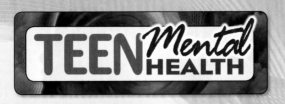

Teens and Eating Disorders

Don Nardo

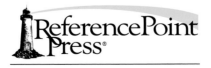

San Diego, CA

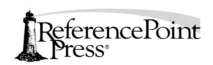

For more information, contact:
ReferencePoint Press, Inc.
PO Box 27779
San Diego, CA 92198
www. ReferencePointPress.com

LIBRARY OF CONGRESS CATALOGING-IN-PUBLICATION DATA

Name: Nardo, Don, 1947– author.
Title: Teens and eating disorders/by Don Nardo.
Description: San Diego, CA: ReferencePoint Press, Inc., 2017. | Series: Teen mental health series | Audience: Grade 9 to 12. | Includes bibliographical references and index.
Identifiers: LCCN 2016026530 (print) | LCCN 2016027158 (ebook) | ISBN 9781682821220 (hardback) | ISBN 9781682821237 (eBook)
Subjects: LCSH: Eating disorders in children. | Eating disorders in children--Treatment.
Classification: LCC RJ506.E18 N37 2017 (print) | LCC RJ506.E18 (ebook) | DDC 618.92/8526--dc23
LC record available at https://lccn.loc.gov/2016026530

CONTENTS

Introduction   4
   "The Monster Inside Me"

Chapter One   8
   What Are Eating Disorders?

Chapter Two   22
   What Causes Eating Disorders?

Chapter Three   37
   What Is It Like to Live with an Eating Disorder?

Chapter Four   51
   Can Eating Disorders Be Treated or Cured?

Source Notes   65

Recognizing Signs of Trouble   69

Organizations to Contact   70

For Further Research   73

Index   75

Picture Credits   79

About the Author   80

"The Monster Inside Me"

"**W**hen I look back on my journey, I'm in awe of how my eating disorder changed my life," says Julie Saunders, now in her twenties. An eating disorder is a serious medical condition in which a person's normal, healthy eating habits have been disrupted, with decidedly *un*healthy results. In telling her painful story, Saunders points out that this disruption was not something she expected, or even considered at all, before it occurred. "For 18 years I never once thought about what I was eating," she explains. Neither did she pay much attention to her "clothing size, my weight on the scale, and certainly not calories or my exercise. I was as carefree as they come, I was constantly surrounded by friends, laughing until I cried, and eating whenever and whatever I wanted. I couldn't tell you how many calories I ate or what I weighed because that was something that never crossed my mind."[1]

A Shrinking Will to Live

But then, seemingly out of nowhere, one incident changed everything. Often called the trigger, or ignition switch, that sets an eating disorder in motion, in Saunders's case it was a negative remark someone made about her weight. In and of itself, Saunders says, such a comment might seem small, even trivial. Yet, she adds with a touch of regret, it "changed my life forever." In the space of only a few months, she went from a happy and outgoing individual "to the girl who hid herself from the world."[2]

Indeed, the eating disorder seemed to take over Saunders's life. She says that she began measuring her self-worth by the number of calories she consumed and the number of pounds registering on her scale. Moreover, she viewed any increases in her weight, even tiny ones, not only as something bad but also as the result of her own inadequacies. "I thought I wasn't trying hard enough," she recalls. So she constantly tried harder to keep from gaining weight, including working out "for countless hours every day."[3]

The result was that Saunders started losing weight at what she calls "an alarming rate." At the same time, her desire to live shrank along with her body. "Along the way I also lost all of my friends," she continues. "I missed out on family events and spending time with my loved ones because I was afraid of being tempted with food, afraid of my secret being exposed."[4]

> "I cried when I thought of food and berated myself for eating. I was a shell of who I once was."[5]
>
> —Eating disorder sufferer Julie Saunders

A Shell of Her Former Self

Saunders's weight loss and emotional fears and discomfort were not the only adverse effects of the eating disorder that had taken control of her life. "My hair fell out," she remembers. In addition, she often felt dizzy and her clothes no longer fit right. "My eyes were dark holes," her painful testimony goes on.

> I cried when I thought of food and berated myself for eating. I was a shell of who I once was. Every day I thought to myself that I couldn't live this way forever, but the alternative was me gaining weight, and at the time, that was even worse than being consumed by the monster inside me that was my eating disorder.[5]

Making matters worse, Saunders found that more comments by the people in her life about her changing weight gave her even more incentive to keep losing. "The more weight I lost," she says, "the more compliments I received. Even at times when I knew I

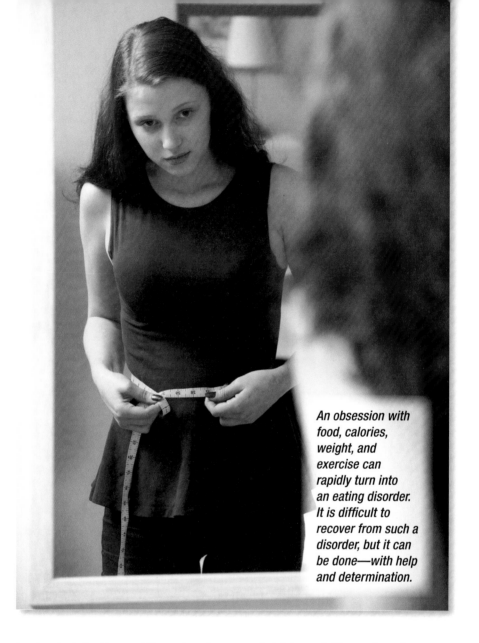

An obsession with food, calories, weight, and exercise can rapidly turn into an eating disorder. It is difficult to recover from such a disorder, but it can be done—with help and determination.

looked sick, they still praised my weight loss." Saunders is convinced that such inadvertently harmful social input is one reason "why people fail to get the help they need. When your peers are condoning your habits, you think you're fine."[6]

Getting Her Life Back

It took Saunders a long time to realize that her insidious condition had ruined her life. "An eating disorder is a slow death, an unspoken suicide," she says. "Now I see life differently. I regained my health and saved my life. I go out with my friends and no longer skip out on family events." She cheerfully adds that her "hair is long and healthy"[7] and that she has learned to smile again.

Most importantly, Saunders has managed to get her eating habits and the manner in which she views food and the act of eating itself under control. "I eat to fuel my body," she says proudly. "I exercise a healthy amount and if I'm not up to working out, then I choose not to. I find happiness in the smallest things that I was blind to before. I think what's most important is that I don't feel guilty for being happy, for making mistakes and being human."[8]

Much to her relief, Saunders learned that although no cure yet exists for eating disorders, they *can* be managed and brought under control. Thus, she says, having this sort of condition does not have to be a death sentence. "Recovery isn't something that is easy," she admits. "It isn't something that happens over night. It takes determination and hard work. At every meal you have to make the choice to choose recovery over your disordered eating thoughts. Recovery enabled me to find strength within myself and to find my voice that my eating disorder silenced."[9]

> "Recovery enabled me to find strength within myself and to find my voice that my eating disorder silenced."[9]
>
> —Julie Saunders

A much more confident Saunders says that she now looks forward to her future, one she feels is filled with hope. Smiling, she concludes that learning to manage her eating disorder "gave me back my life."[10]

CHAPTER ONE

What Are Eating Disorders?

E ating disorders are medical conditions characterized by harm-ful eating habits and patterns. In most cases, individuals with eating disorders eat either too much or too little and as a result suffer from various physical, emotional, and even social problems. The seriousness of these problems cannot be overstated. Indeed, according to the National Eating Disorders Association (NEDA),

> Eating disorders are real, complex, and devastating con-ditions that can have serious consequences for health, productivity, and relationships. They are not a fad, phase or lifestyle choice. Eating disorders are serious, potentially life-threatening conditions that affect a person's emotional and physical health. People struggling with an eating dis-order need to seek professional help. The earlier a person with an eating disorder seeks treatment, the greater the likelihood of physical and emotional recovery.[11]

The Grim Statistics

Aside from the physical, emotional, and other effects of eating disorders, these conditions are serious partly because they are widespread, affecting people of both genders, all ages, and all social and economic classes. NEDA estimates that in the United States alone, 20 million women and 10 million men suffer from one of these disorders. That is nearly 10 percent of the population of the country.

Furthermore, in many cases such conditions begin in childhood or adolescence, so teens and twenty-somethings are major risk groups for developing them. The National Association of Anorexia Nervosa and Associated Disorders (ANAD) reports that 95 percent of those who have eating disorders are between the ages of twelve and twenty-six. Of these cases, moreover, 86 percent develop by age twenty, and 43 percent emerge between the ages of sixteen and twenty alone. This suggests that people in their late teens are most at risk for developing eating disorders.

An unknown proportion of these youthful cases of eating disorders do not become seriously debilitating. But many other cases *do* end up disrupting sufferers' lives in diverse ways. According to the National Institute of Mental Health (NIMH), which closely monitors and studies eating disorders, at least 2.7 percent of young people between the ages of thirteen and eighteen develop severe eating disorders that remain lifetime problems.

> "Eating disorders are serious, potentially life-threatening conditions that affect a person's emotional and physical health."[11]
>
> —The National Eating Disorders Association

Among these serious health problems, ANAD states, close to half of the individuals with eating disorders suffer from clinical depression to some degree. Moreover, more than half of teenage girls and nearly one-third of teenage boys regularly employ unhealthy weight control behaviors. These include forced vomiting, fasting too often, smoking cigarettes, skipping too many meals, and taking large doses of laxatives. Other negative outcomes that can occur later include muscle and/or joint pain, insomnia or sleep apnea, type 2 diabetes, and heart disease. Making matters worse, the experts point out, only one out of ten people with eating disorders actually ends up receiving treatment. Also, just 35 percent of people who manage to get treated do so at a facility that specializes in eating disorders.

Still more grim statistics show that an alarming number of eating disorder cases are ultimately fatal. ANAD reports that these detrimental conditions have the highest mortality, or death, rate of any mental illness. For example, the mortality rate for perhaps the best-known eating disorder—anorexia—is twelve times higher than the death rate for all causes of death for females aged fifteen to twenty-four. Moreover, 5 to 10 percent of anorexics die within ten years of developing the illness, and 18 to 20 percent of anorexics die after suffering from the disorder for twenty years.

The Gateway

Leading health experts and organizations recognize two other major eating disorders besides anorexia. These are binge eating and bulimia. Each of these harmful conditions has typical, recognizable symptoms—or signs and patterns of behavior—that distinguish it from other illnesses. Yet the three main eating disorders are not unrelated conditions. In fact, they are closely related because each is a component of a larger, overarching pattern of disordered behaviors related to food and eating. For instance, all three are either involved with or are a reaction to the misuse of food and its often damaging consequences.

For these reasons, binge eaters, bulimics, and anorexics frequently exhibit some, or even several, of the same symptoms and behaviors. Furthermore, ample evidence shows that one of the three disorders often leads to another in a disturbing progression.

With few exceptions, the first stage of that unhealthy progression is binge eating. Experts have fairly regularly changed the disorder's official name, referring to it as compulsive overeating, emotional eating, and food addiction, among other terms. Whatever one chooses to call it, binge eating disorder is often the gateway to the even more severe disorders anorexia and bulimia. Thus, all bulimics and anorexics either start out as binge eaters or at least sometimes engage in binge eating behavior.

The Symptoms of Binge Eating

Experts point out that binge eating is the most common eating disorder in the United States. NEDA states that it affects about 3.5 percent of adult women, 2 percent of adult men, and up to 1.6 percent of teenagers. As is true of other eating disorders, anyone,

Common Symptoms of Anorexia, Bulimia, and Binge Eating

The three most common eating disorders—anorexia, bulimia, and binge eating—all involve potentially grave problems with eating behavior and weight control. Extreme weight loss, secretive eating habits, and unrelenting worry about one's own body weight or shape are common signs of an eating disorder.

Anorexia

Symptoms include:

- Extremely restricted eating
- Extreme thinness (emaciation)
- A relentless pursuit of thinness and unwillingness to maintain a normal or healthy weight
- Intense fear of gaining weight
- Distorted body image, a self--esteem that is heavily influenced by perceptions of body weight and shape, or a denial of the seriousness of low body weight

Other symptoms may develop over time, including:

- Thinning of the bones (osteopenia or osteoporosis)
- Mild anemia and muscle wasting and weakness
- Brittle hair and nails
- Dry and yellowish skin
- Growth of fine hair all over the body (lanugo)
- Severe constipation
- Low blood pressure, slowed breathing and pulse
- Damage to the structure and function of the heart
- Brain damage
- Multiorgan failure
- Drop in internal body temperature, causing a person to feel cold all the time
- Lethargy, sluggishness, or feeling tired all the time
- Infertility

Bulimia

Symptoms include:

- Chronically inflamed and sore throat
- Swollen salivary glands in the neck and jaw area
- Worn tooth enamel and increasingly sensitive and decaying teeth as a result of exposure to stomach acid
- Acid reflux disorder and other gastrointestinal problems
- Intestinal distress and irritation from laxatives
- Severe dehydration from purging of fluids
- Electrolyte imbalance (too low or too high levels of sodium, calcium, potassium, and other minerals) which can lead to stroke or heart attack

Binge Eating

Symptoms include:

- Eating unusually large amounts of food in a specific amount of time
- Eating even when you're full or not hungry
- Eating fast during binge episodes
- Eating until you're uncomfortably full
- Eating alone or in secret to avoid embarrassment
- Feeling distressed, ashamed, or guilty about your eating
- Frequently dieting, possibly without weight loss

Source: National Institute of Mental Health. "Eating Disorders: About More than Food." February 2016. www.nimh.gov.

regardless of race, religion, or economic level, can become a binge eater.

As its name suggests, binge eating is characterized by a person's consuming abnormally large amounts of food in a single sitting. The general tendency is for the person to feast on large amounts of highly caloric and fattening foods. Often these include doughnuts, potato chips, ice cream, pie, cake, cookies, cheeseburgers, and so forth. However, it is not uncommon for binge eaters to eat healthy foods, such as fruits, vegetables, and lean meats, instead of or in addition to pastries, snack foods, and the like.

Whatever a binge eater's choices of food may be, the key behavior is consuming far more than is healthy at one time. As an expert on the disorder, Dr. John M. Grohol, puts it, "The specific type of food doesn't matter. What matters is the sheer amount of food consumed in one sitting."[12] It is not unusual, for example, for a person to eat an entire cake or pie, plus a gallon of ice cream, in the course of ten or fifteen minutes. Indeed, some binge eaters admit to taking in up to ten thousand calories in a single binge— roughly the amount an average person eats in four days.

What is more, most binge eaters engage in the behavior fairly often. According to Grohol, even those with the mildest cases of the condition tend to binge from one to three times per week. Moderate bingeing behavior, he says, involves four to seven episodes per week; and severe cases witness from eight to fourteen binges per week. In addition, Grohol explains, during a binge the sufferer typically displays such abnormal behaviors as "eating much more rapidly than normal, eating until feeling uncomfortably full, eating large amounts of food when not feeling physically hungry," and "eating alone because of feeling embarrassed by how much one is eating."[13]

A Preoccupation with Food

As a result of these seemingly frenzied episodes of overeating, it is common for binge eaters to become overweight to one degree or another. Unhappy with such weight gain, many of these individuals stop bingeing for a few weeks or more in hopes of losing

Eating Disorders Are Finally on the Public Radar

For eating disorders, 1982 proved to be a milestone year. Before that time, the vast majority of people had never heard of these conditions, and even many doctors were only marginally aware of them. In part, this was because before that time research into those disorders had been on a small scale. Perhaps more importantly, no high profile public case of an eating disorder had previously drawn large-scale media attention. The great turning point that year was the publication of a book by Cherry Boone O'Neill, the daughter of well-known singer and actor Pat Boone. Titled *Starving for Attention,* the book quickly became a best seller. In it, O'Neill explained that she had battled with anorexia and had eventually ended up in a hospital weighing a mere eighty pounds. With the help of dedicated doctors, her family, and friends, she said, she managed to recover and to adopt healthy eating habits once again. This frank account of a young woman struggling against the ravages of anorexia touched a nerve with the American public. O'Neill also made the rounds of television and radio talk shows. In those programs that were open to phone calls, a number of young women called in to say that they too suffered from anorexia. Thereafter, anorexia and other eating disorders were squarely on the radar of both the health care community and the general public.

the excess weight. Such a person might go on a reducing diet or simply eat normal amounts of food.

This attempt to counteract the negative effects of regular bingeing nearly always fails. After losing some or all of the weight, the person almost inevitably returns to bingeing. One common result of this extreme yo-yo succession of alternating behaviors is repeated weight changes of ten to twenty pounds or more. Some sufferers eventually become exhausted by the cycle of gaining and losing, give up on dieting, and allow themselves to become obese, or significantly overweight. (Doctors say that a person is obese if he or she exhibits a body mass index of 30 or more. Body mass index is a weight calculation based on the ratio of a person's height and weight. The range considered to be normal for adults is 18.5 to 24.9. Because teenagers are still growing and changing, there is no standard range of body mass index for this group.)

Thus, a person who once had an average, normal, healthy body with little or no excess weight can, through binge eating, become perpetually overweight or even obese. Mention of that person's once normal condition naturally brings up the question of the age at which binge eating most often takes hold. Studies reveal that the disorder and its negative behaviors most often begin fairly early in life.

> "[Food] signified love and hate. It brought me up and then down. It was my best friend and my worst enemy."[14]
>
> —Eating disorder sufferer Chevese

Typical is the story of a binge eater who calls herself Chevese. "Sometime between the ages of five and seven," she says, "I discovered the power of food. I discovered I wanted more of it than I was permitted to have, that it was a restricted temptation, and I thought about it a lot. It calmed and shamed me at the same time. It signified love and hate. It brought me up and then down. It was my best friend and my worst enemy."[14]

As a child, Chevese explains, she liked playing with her friends, just as most children do. However, she would frequently cut playtimes short in order to go home and enjoy some snacks in her parents' kitchen. She would also have snacks at her friends' houses whenever possible. "I did not like to ask for food," she says. "I was ashamed, even at an early age, of my preoccupation [with food]."[15]

Without attempting to pinpoint the causes of that strong fixation with food, Chevese does remember that her mother may well have had an eating disorder herself. She "insisted that I 'eat healthy' and taught me to distinguish between 'good' and 'bad' food early in my childhood," Chevese states. Yet her mother "had her own problems with food. For her, it was love, but it was also a source of control. She learned during her own difficult childhood and teenage years that she had power over food and herself if she denied hunger. She was probably anorexic, although she was never officially diagnosed or treated."[16]

A Strong Element of Shame

Chevese's abnormal preoccupation with food never progressed beyond her periodic binges. She did not move further along in the eating disorders spectrum and take what is potentially the next, even more harmful step. Namely, she did not regularly rid herself of the large amounts of food she consumed. If she had deliberately vomited out most of what she had eaten, she would have become what health experts designate as a bulimic.

Thus, those individuals who suffer from bulimia typically start out as binge eaters. Like the latter, bulimics habitually go on benders in which they take in huge amounts of food. But unlike binge eaters, bulimics usually purge, or vomit out, most or all of that excess food. The word *usually* must be emphasized here because some bulimics also rid themselves of the food by using laxatives and/or diuretics, medications that make them go to the bathroom.

People who suffer from bulimia normally binge and purge at least once a week, according to the Canadian National Eating Disorders Information Centre (NEDIC). Some bulimics do so two or more times per week. Often the behavior becomes part of a debilitating cycle, as in the case of a bulimic named Sara. "When I had been heavier," she recalls,

> I had been deemed "unlovable." This is when I started seriously making myself sick [i.e., vomiting]. Every time I ate or drank I would be sick. I would also "compete" with myself to see how long I could go without eating. Each day I would wake up, determined to beat my record from the day before. If I succeeded I would reward myself with a bowl of cereal, which more often than not, would lead into a binge and purge because I had starved myself the entire day.[17]

Moreover, like other bulimics, Sara always engaged in this characteristic behavior in secret. Sufferers are aware that what they are doing is out of control and will be viewed as abnormal by their family and friends, so there is a strong element of shame involved. As a result, the number of bulimics in society may well be higher than the number of cases reported to medical authorities.

The Signs and Dangers of Bulimia

If educated to do so, the families and friends of bulimics can look for a number of characteristics or common symptoms of the condition. Indeed, according to Eating Disorder Hope, a group dedicated to eradicating these disorders, sufferers frequently "reveal several signs and symptoms, many of which are the direct result of self-induced vomiting or other forms of purging, especially if the binge/purge cycle is repeated several times a week and/or day."[18]

One of the leading symptoms of bulimia, medical experts say, is regular fluctuations in a person's weight. These changes occur because the sufferer will sometimes gain weight due to his or her food binges. Other times that individual will exhibit lower-than-normal body weight as a result of repeated vomiting episodes. Other telltale signs of bulimia are frequent use of the bathroom after meals, continually smelling like vomit, broken blood vessels in the eyes (from the strain of heavy vomiting), enlarged glands in the neck area (another result of constant vomiting), and the disappearance of large amounts of food from the household.

If these signs of the ailment are ignored and it progresses without any intervention, the bulimic can suffer from one or more serious conditions. Common, for instance, are small cuts in the lining of the mouth or throat, caused by repeated vomiting. Also typical are swelling of the esophagus and infertility. In addition, constant vomiting often causes dehydration, as do excessive exercise and misuse of laxatives and diuretics—all of which are also associated with bulimia. "These types of purging can lead to imbalances in essential body minerals and salts, which can cause cardiac arrest and/or stroke,"[19] a spokesperson for NEDIC explains.

A Distortion of Body Image

Still another danger that bulimics face on a regular basis is the chance they will eventually feel their purging is not controlling their weight well enough. Some of those who come to this conclusion

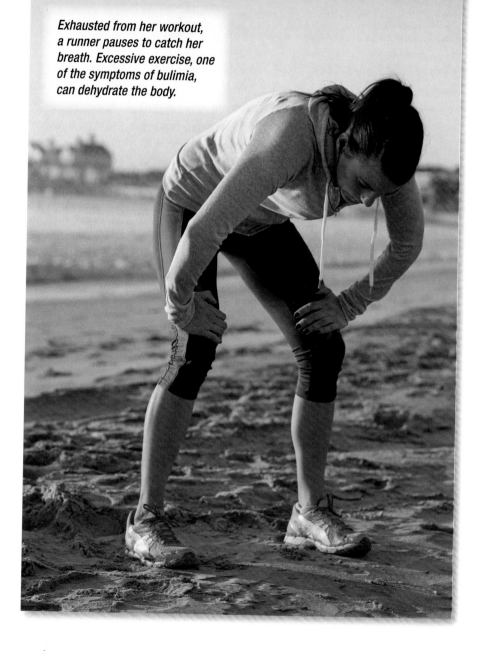

Exhausted from her workout, a runner pauses to catch her breath. Excessive exercise, one of the symptoms of bulimia, can dehydrate the body.

end up crossing a sort of invisible line. From a health perspective, it marks the boundary between bulimia and potentially the most damaging eating disorder of all—anorexia.

Like sufferers of binge eating and bulimia, anorexics usually start out experiencing problems with excess weight. Some gain only a few pounds, but others may initially become obese. Either way, they develop an intense dread of becoming or remaining fat, and their reaction is extreme. More often than not, they go on

Eating Disorders Among Young Men

"Prevalence figures for males with eating disorders are somewhat elusive." states NEDA. "In the past, eating disorders have been characterized as 'women's problems' and men have been stigmatized from coming forward or have been unaware that they could have an eating disorder." NEDA and other organizations that study eating disorders say that much additional research is needed before a meaningful picture of how these conditions affect men emerges. But some limited studies have been conducted and have yielded some preliminary data. First, it appears that about 10 million males in the United States at any given time will develop an eating disorder. Also a study of 1,383 teenagers found that about 1.2 percent of boys aged fourteen had an eating disorder, and roughly 2.6 percent of young men aged seventeen had such a condition. That percentage increased to 2.9 for those males turning from age nineteen to age twenty. A different study—this one involving 2,822 college students—showed that 3.6 percent of young men already suffered from binge eating, bulimia, or anorexia. (The study found that the percentage of females with eating disorders was about three times that of the males.) Interestingly, other studies found that among males in their teens and twenties, those who were gay were three times more likely to suffer from an eating disorder than those who were straight.

National Eating Disorders Association, "Research on Males and Eating Disorders." www.nationaleatingdisorders.org.

reducing diets that involve self-starvation. According to ANAD, anorexia typically features a

> relentless pursuit of thinness and unwillingness to maintain a normal or healthy weight, a distortion of body image and intense fear of gaining weight, a lack of menstruation among girls and women, and extremely disturbed eating behavior. . . . Many people with anorexia see themselves as overweight, even when they are starved or are clearly malnourished. Eating, food and weight control become obsessions. A person with anorexia typically weighs herself or himself repeatedly, portions food carefully, and eats only very small quantities of only certain foods.[20]

An anorexic who calls herself Zivile states, "I started refusing everything except for carrots and apples. It was my daily bread. Not surprisingly, very soon I weighed less and less." Not knowing any better, she says, she "thought that not eating normally was something that expressed my individuality. I thought that eating carrots and apples helped to increase my self-discipline and persistence in my schoolwork."[21]

Unhealthy Symptoms and Complications

As the illness came to increasingly control her life, Zivile displayed several classic symptoms of anorexia, some of which tend to be interrelated. They included eating far less than was healthy, becoming abnormally thin, constantly pursuing even more thinness, and fearing the very idea of gaining weight. She also displayed distorted body image; specifically seeing herself as heavier than she actually was. In addition, she exhibited serious low self-esteem based on her misguided perception that she was overweight.

Integral to the distorted and misguided aspects of an anorexic's range of symptoms is a lack of awareness that she or he suffers from the disorder. One sufferer, Kristine, later recalled, "My malnourished and young adolescent mind could not comprehend the seriousness of this illness."[22] Other anorexics realize their disorder exists but fail to grasp the degree of danger involved. According to a young woman who calls herself Jasmine,

> "Many people with anorexia see themselves as overweight, even when they are starved or are clearly malnourished."[20]
>
> —The National Association of Anorexia Nervosa and Associated Disorders

At first, no one addressed my weight loss, which led me to believe it wasn't noticeable. I strove to lose more and practically lived on the scale. The scale served as a sanctuary, yet it could also be a tormentor. I felt proud of my motivation and accomplishment when I lost a pound and I punished myself if I didn't. While I was aware that I had some kind of a problem, I didn't realize its severity and was not ready to seek help.[23]

Still another common complication of anorexia involves occasionally slipping into behaviors associated with other eating disorders. On the one hand, an anorexic repeatedly rejects food, becoming thinner and thinner. On the other, however, these sufferers still strongly desire food, even if they try to convince themselves that they do not. The result of this ongoing battle within an anorexic's own mind is that she or he may now and then go on a classic binge. When this happens, the individual will pack away large amounts of highly caloric foods, such as cookies, pie, cake, or ice cream. Then, inevitably, the person will regret doing so and will try to counteract the mistake by drastic dieting or purging. Or she or he may load up on laxatives and diuretics in a desperate attempt to force the extra food out of the body. Clearly, this cycle of starving, bingeing, and purging, followed by more starving is very unhealthy for anyone's body.

> "I felt proud of my motivation and accomplishment when I lost a pound and I punished myself if I didn't."[23]
>
> —Eating disorder sufferer Jasmine

Anorexia's Unhealthy Effects

In fact, doctors and other health professionals recognize numerous potentially harmful outcomes of anorexia, which vary in number and kind from one sufferer to another. One of the most common of these problems is osteoporosis, which is a thinning of the bones caused by taking in too little calcium and other nutrients. Similarly, anorexics typically experience some degree of anemia—a lack of healthy red blood cells—which can be caused by poor nutrition.

Among the other unhealthy effects of anorexia are constipation, which can be severe and painful at times; brittle nails and hair; sluggishness or feeling tired most of the time; weakness in muscles throughout the body; and for women with the disorder, a lack of fertility, or the inability to conceive children. Many anorexics also develop low blood pressure and/or slowed breathing and pulse. Over time these can damage the heart's structure and function, which is why the risk of heart attack is particularly high for sufferers of anorexia. Finally, for severe, prolonged cases

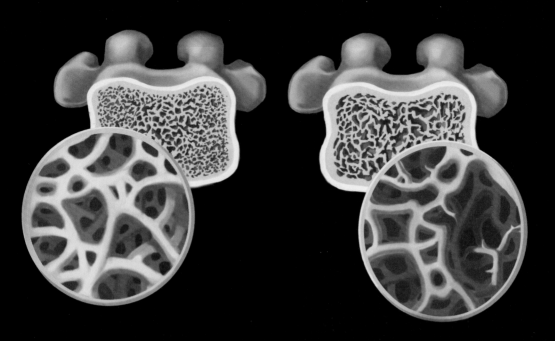

By starving their bodies of needed nutrients, anorexics set themselves up for developing osteoporosis. The inside of a normal bone (left) has a honeycomb pattern. The inside of a bone with osteoporosis (right) has larger spaces, reflecting the loss of bone density and strength.

of anorexia, the risk of multiorgan failure and death significantly increases.

Some anorexics remain stubborn and refuse to face the fact that these physical problems are serious or even that they are related to an eating disorder. This denial of the condition's very existence is perhaps the most dangerous of the disease's negative effects. Years after learning to manage her anorexia, Jasmine unhappily remembered her toughest moments, saying,

> The doctors continued to tell me it was either go into treatment or die within the next few months due to my low weight and dangerously low heart rate. The scary thing is that I was so sick that I actually considered holding onto my eating disorder. I was so afraid and resistant to change my rigid behaviors that I was willing to die just to keep things the same. Now I realize how sick I actually was.[24]

CHAPTER TWO

What Causes Eating Disorders?

The causes of eating disorders are often diverse and complex, says clinical psychologist Deborah A. Russo. Not surprisingly, therefore, those causes "aren't always understood by parents or children and can be hard to detect," she explains.

> The typical symptoms for a child with an eating disorder are often different from adolescents and adults. For instance, we may not directly see or hear signs of a preoccupation with body weight and shape. . . . Hence, many will not meet the full criteria for diagnosing a specific eating disorder and therefore not be taken seriously enough for proper intervention. Diagnosis can be tricky.[25]

In addition to the difficulty in diagnosing eating disorders in some cases, experts sometimes disagree over how influential some factors are in causing these conditions. However, health care professionals and organizations that study eating disorders agree on one central point. Namely, no single, primary factor causes someone to develop these illnesses. Rather, a combination of factors—whether personal, medical, social, or otherwise—is typically involved, and each of those factors affects different people in different ways.

Moreover, the manner in which individuals react to various social pressures varies widely. Some young people learn healthy ways of dealing with changing family and peer relationships, for example, which may make them less likely to develop an eating disorder. Other young people may have more difficulty in dealing with the wide range of "intense . . . socio-cultural pressures"[26] they will inevitably experience in their lives, as Russo puts it. These individuals, she points out, have the highest risk of developing binge eating, bulimia, or anorexia.

Depression and Eating Disorders

In looking for the root causes of eating disorders, experts often begin by studying "the personalities, genetics, environments, and biochemistry of people with these illnesses,"[27] according to California's Palo Alto Medical Foundation. These factors differ for every individual and are crucial in the development of one of the leading causes of eating disorders—depression.

Roughly 5 percent of children and adolescents in the United States suffer from clinical depression at any given moment in time, says the American Academy of Child and Adolescent Psychiatry. Although it is normal to feel sad or gloomy at times, clinical depression is a mental state in which an individual is overwhelmed by feelings of hopelessness and commonly comes to see life itself as meaningless and no longer worth living. According to the academy, major signs of this serious type of depression include a decreased interest in common activities, persistent feelings of low energy and social isolation, low self-esteem, constant guilt over minor matters, extreme fear of rejection or failure, difficulty in forming and maintaining relationships, poor performance in school, frequent headaches, and major changes in sleeping and/or eating habits.

That last symptom of depression—changes in eating habits—is key to understanding one widespread cause of eating disorders. Bulimia sufferer Sara suffered from depression, which her doctors pinpointed as a major factor in her development of an eating disorder. When she was twenty-two, she recalls, she

> had just graduated from university. Society was expecting me to "go out and get a job." Along with a job, I was supposed to get an income, a place to live and to support myself completely independently for the first time in my life.

23

I was terrified. At this very time I was busy feeling rejected and worthless. A serious boyfriend had dumped me, for the second time in my life. It was not a great phase for me. I sank into a very depressive-like state.[28]

While in that state, Sara rarely ate any food; thus, she started to lose weight. "I didn't even realize at first that I was getting smaller," she says. But her friends and family did notice her weight loss. "Everyone kept telling me how great I looked." At that point, Sara remembers, she decided that she would never gain the weight back. That way, she reasoned, she was sure to feel better about herself. Rejecting food on a regular basis "was not only a way to control my weight," she says, "it was [also] a way to control my emotions."[29] Unfortunately for Sara, when she continued to eat very little food, her body reacted by craving food all the more. In turn, that triggered her destructive cycle of bingeing and purging.

The Issue of Self-Esteem

Evidence shows that other crucial personal factors in the development of eating disorders are low self-esteem and poor body image. Young people who suffer from these inward-looking perceptions may see themselves as unattractive, unintelligent, inept, untalented, and/or worthless. They are likely to feel inadequate and unable to measure up to average social standards. They may then turn to coping mechanisms, or ways to compensate for supposed failings. One of those mechanisms can be overeating because food may become a sort of crutch, something to make them feel better for at least a little while.

According to Eating Disorders Victoria, an Australian group that provides people with helpful information about these conditions, low self-esteem and poor body image are connected. Therefore, they can work together in making someone abuse food on a regular basis. Low self-esteem, the group's website states, often "creates and feeds perceptions of poor body image. Low self esteem naturally leads to negative perceptions of one's physical appearance."[30]

Who Is Most at Risk for Developing an Eating Disorder?

No one knows for sure why some people develop an eating disorder and others do not. However, medical experts have identified certain causes and risk factors that increase the likelihood of developing an eating disorder. Genetics is one possible cause: Individuals who have parents or siblings with an eating disorder might have a gene that heightens the risk of developing the disorder. Age is another possible factor: Evidence suggests that people in their teens and early twenties have a higher risk of developing eating disorders than people in other age groups.

Causes

The exact cause of eating disorders is unknown. As with other mental illnesses, there may be many causes, such as:

Genetics. Certain people may have genes that increase their risk of developing eating disorders. People with first-degree relatives—siblings or parents—with an eating disorder may be more likely to develop an eating disorder, too.

Psychological and emotional health. People with eating disorders may have psychological and emotional problems that contribute to the disorder. They may have low self-esteem, perfectionism, impulsive behavior, and troubled relationships.

Society. Success and worth are often equated with being thin in popular culture. Peer pressure and what people see in the media may fuel this desire to be thin.

Risk factors

Certain situations and events might increase the risk of developing an eating disorder. These factors might include:

Being female. Teenage girls and young women are more likely than teenage boys and young men to have anorexia or bulimia, but males can have eating disorders, too.

Age. Although eating disorders can occur across a broad age range—including childhood, the teenage years, and older adulthood—they are much more common during the teens and early twenties.

Family history. Eating disorders are significantly more likely to occur in people who have parents or siblings who've had an eating disorder.

Mental health disorders. People with depression, anxiety disorder, or obsessive-compulsive disorder are more likely to have an eating disorder.

Dieting. People who lose weight are often reinforced by positive comments from others and by their changing appearance. This may cause some people to take dieting too far, leading to an eating disorder.

Stress. Whether it's heading off to college, moving, landing a new job, or a family or relationship issue, change can bring stress, which may increase the risk of an eating disorder.

Sports, work, and artistic activities. Athletes, actors, dancers, and models may be at higher risk for eating disorders. Coaches and parents may unwittingly contribute to eating disorders by encouraging young athletes to lose weight.

Source: The Mayo Clinic, "Eating Disorders: Symptoms and Causes," February 12, 2016. www.mayoclinic.org.

Furthermore, experts on eating disorders say, one's distorted body image can improve only when one's self-esteem becomes stronger. "Self esteem determines how a person lives," Eating Disorders Victoria explains. One's feelings of self-esteem also affect how he or she "talks, handles relationships, chooses career paths, and creates lifestyles. Low self esteem is a major risk factor in the development of an eating disorder."[31]

School-Related Pressures

School-related pressures are another factor in the development of eating disorders among young people. It is not unusual, for instance, for academic pressures to cause an adolescent to gain a few pounds. In a written recollection titled "Picture Perfect Memories," a young woman named Samantha tells how she developed an eating disorder in her quest to achieve perfection—both as a daughter and a student. Of her parents, she says,

> They had high academic expectations for me; so straight As were a must, not a goal. Getting below an A on a test was shameful, embarrassing. I wanted to be the perfect daughter. So when my mom started a new diet my sophomore year, I joined in. For a few weeks, it was okay. Disordered? Probably. But mostly okay. But I fell down the slippery slope that is anorexia all too easily. Counting calories and cutting back on foods I considered "bad" gave me a power trip; ignoring hunger cues made me feel so in control of everything.[32]

Student athletes are also vulnerable to developing eating disorders. They often feel intense pressure—sometimes from parents and coaches and sometimes self-imposed—to either lose or gain weight to make the team. Responding to this pressure, some young athletes resort to unhealthy diets and develop an obsession with their weight. This, in turn, can develop into an eating disorder. Female figure skaters and gymnasts are among the young athletes who are prone to eating disorders because they are expected to be slim. Any extra weight is considered undesirable and must be shed. Yet these young female athletes are not the only ones to experience such pressures.

Studies show that young male athletes are also vulnerable to eating disorders. In sports like swimming, bodybuilding, and gymnastics, NEDA estimates that as many as a third of male athletes develop eating disorders. Particularly vulnerable are the male athletes in so-called weight-class sports, such as wrestling and rowing. Evidence shows that wrestlers sometimes drop weight quickly, partly by eating and drinking less than normal, as well as by taking laxatives and diuretics.

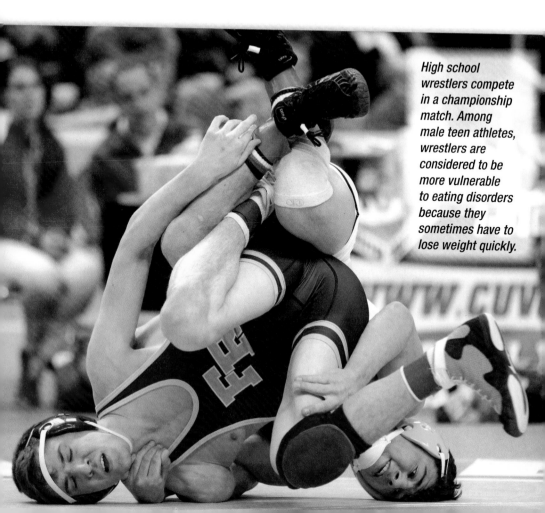

High school wrestlers compete in a championship match. Among male teen athletes, wrestlers are considered to be more vulnerable to eating disorders because they sometimes have to lose weight quickly.

Bullying and Eating Disorders

Experts on eating disorders agree that bullying can contribute to the development of these conditions. "Bullying used to be confined to the schoolyard," states Eating Disorder Hope, an organization that provides information and useful resources to people suffering from those illnesses. But the situation has changed. Eating Disorder Hope contends that

> today, bullying is evidenced in every segment of society in every possible venue from professional sports events to city transit buses. Relational bullying is escalating at a rapid rate throughout our country. This is bullying that transpires within female friendships. It starts very young, as early as second and third grade, and can have profoundly negative long-term consequences such as eating disorders.
>
> The problem is that a girl who is only eight or ten years old lacks the emotional maturity to understand what is happening to her. She may well believe the bullies who call her fat, or stupid, or worthless. If she does believe it, her self-esteem may become badly impaired. This sort of cruelty sometimes transpires for years, doing more and more damage and eventually leading to depression and anxiety. "If she does not possess healthy coping skills or a positive support system at home," Eating Disorder Hope states, "this can eventually result in an eating disorder."

Eating Disorder Hope, "Teen Relational Bullying: Verbal Abuse That Can Trigger Eating Disorders." www.eating disorderhope.com.

Another school-related pressure that can factor into the development of an eating disorder is bullying, which remains common in most American schools. A young woman named Jackie DiVito remembers being made fun of in grade school because she was overly plump. "I was bullied so badly about my looks," she recalls, "that when I was in seventh grade I actually had to switch schools." The bullying did not end there for her, however. "I was bullied in middle school and high school," she says, "and by age seventeen I had a full-blown eating disorder."[33]

Social Trends and the Media

Experts say that the effects of parental and school pressures in the development of eating disorders are frequently reinforced by social trends and images portrayed in the media. For example, there has long been a strong emphasis on physical thinness in clothing sales and print ads for all manner of products as well as television shows and movies. Young women are particularly targeted and susceptible to relentless images of overly skinny models and actresses.

This glorification of bodily thinness was not always in vogue. In the 1940s, 1950s, and well into the 1960s—curvy, even somewhat plump actresses like Marilyn Monroe, Jane Russell, and Jayne Mansfield were seen to possess ideal feminine forms. The image of the skinny-as-a-rail model or actress began to take firm hold in the 1970s and thereafter became the norm. As recently as 2016, for example, the well-known Italian fashion brand Gucci ran an online video ad featuring a very thin model. An influential fashion industry watchdog group, the Advertising Standards Authority, called the ad irresponsible because it used a model whose body was disproportionate, overly thin, and looked unhealthy.

Further reinforcing this trend was the rise of an enormous diet industry that promoted, and still widely encourages, weight reduction plans of all kinds. Ads for and sales of expensive exercise machines also became common in magazines and television infomercials. Doctors, especially mental health specialists, point out that this continuous emphasis on thinness can sometimes actually damage people's health. Most people who try fad diets in hopes of losing weight do so without sound medical advice. Often they starve themselves to one degree or another. That can trigger food binges, which in turn can lead to bulimia and in some cases anorexia.

The rise of the Internet and social media has also contributed to the spread of eating disorders in recent decades. First, the screen of any computer or handheld tablet is now an easily navigated portal to pro-ana, or pro-anorexia, websites. There are also pro-mia, or pro-bulimia, sites. Many of these online destinations claim that anorexia and bulimia are not illnesses but rather lifestyle choices or harmless fads. Despite warnings from doctors and other medical professionals that such websites are misleading and potentially harmful, they still attract millions of viewers.

Similarly, other forms of social media, including Facebook, Twitter, Tumblr, Instagram, and Pinterest, are sometimes used as platforms on which certain anorexics and bulimics claim they are not sick. Instead, they say, they have made personal lifestyle choices that people should respect. Nevertheless, these same social media outlets have also become platforms for eating disorder sufferers who admit they are ill. Typically these individuals share their personal stories, warn other young people to beware of these conditions, and promote legitimate medical treatments.

Describing social media in general, Claire Mysko, NEDA's head of youth outreach, says, "We live in a culture where eating disorders thrive because of the messages we're exposed to." The various kinds of social media, she warns, can sometimes "heighten that exposure."[34] When employed the wrong way, Mysko adds, social media can amplify unhealthy behaviors associated with eating disorders, such as obsessions with food or thinness.

> "We live in a culture where eating disorders thrive because of the messages we're exposed to."[34]
>
> —Claire Mysko, head of youth outreach for NEDA

Seeking Perfection

One of the most often discussed causes for eating disorders is psychological in nature, or related to how a person's mind perceives the world around her or him. In this case, the person is mentally and emotionally intent on achieving perfection whenever possible. She or he tends to be an overachiever and actually does accomplish a great deal. Yet that is not enough for a perfectionist. In spite of all that earnest effort, he or she may still feel inadequate, even useless.

The term that a number of experts use to denote the attitude of such individuals is *perfectionistic*. "They have unrealistic expectations of themselves and others," says one authority on eating disorders. "In addition, they see the world as black and white, [with] no shades of gray. Everything is either good or bad, a success or a failure, fat or thin. If fat is bad and thin is good, then thinner is better, and thinnest is best, even if thinnest is [ending up weighing] sixty-eight pounds in a hospital bed on life support."[35]

A young former anorexic named Christina knows firsthand how the quest for personal perfection can lead a person into the unhealthy habits linked with eating disorders. "I felt pressured by my family to live up to perfectionistic standards," she recalls.

> For as long as I can remember my family was all about looking good and keeping up with that image, rather than internally feeling good. I remember the first time I ever thought I was ugly. I was dressed for private school in my uniform for the first day of kindergarten, with my hair in a bun on the top of my head. I saw myself in the mirror and I remember feeling less than [happy] because I had to look that way. I also believed that I had fallen short as a person because I was made fun of a lot growing up in school. Between these two pressures that I felt, I developed severe self-esteem issues at an early age. I would think to myself, "Is there something wrong with me?" "Maybe if I can find out and fix whatever is wrong with me, I can take charge and have some form of control in my life, so I can say that I finally feel happy inside."[36]

Young people who tend to be perfectionists and thereby particularly vulnerable to developing eating disorders are often heavily into the arts or athletics. Dancers, who combine artistic talent with intense athleticism, are especially at risk for developing these dangerous medical conditions. Arden Whitehurst, who began dancing early in life, has published a summary of her struggle with anorexia on the Internet, saying in part,

> From the outside I've always had everything going for me. But on the inside I was an anxious child and very much a perfectionist. When I was fourteen I began obsessing

about ballet (even more). I wore myself out and was an anxious mess. I started auditioning for summer programs and saw that everyone was better than me [and] thinner than me. I thought that had to be the difference. They were better because they were thinner. From that point on I was obsessed about the "perfect" ballet body. It became my ideal. I suffered severe depression and anxiety and took a month or so off over the summer. [The] Nutcracker [ballet] came [and] things got worse. I made it through Nutcracker, still hiding my secret. Finally, through a series of events, my secret came out, and doctors' appointments followed. Then at sixteen came the diagnosis—anorexia.[37]

Triggers Set the Ball in Motion

It is sometimes difficult to pinpoint an explicit underlying cause for a particular case of disordered eating. But after devoting much time and effort to searching for a culprit, patients often remember that the bingeing, purging, and/or starvation began shortly after a specific event. That occurrence might or might not have been important or memorable at the time.

Experts call such an isolated event a trigger. According to the organization Anorexia Nervosa and Related Eating Disorders (ANRED), "Of the people who are vulnerable to eating disorders, sometimes all it takes to put the ball in motion is a trigger event that they do not know how to handle." Such a trigger "could be something as seemingly innocuous as teasing or as devastating as rape or incest." Other common triggers that can lead to eating disorders occur "at times of transition, shock, or loss," ANRED explains. They can include "puberty, starting a new school, beginning a new job, death, divorce, marriage, family problems, breakup of an important relationship, critical comments from someone important, graduation into a chaotic, competitive world, and so forth."[38]

Of these triggers, reaching puberty appears to be more common than most in setting eating disorders in motion. Some evidence suggests that young women who transition into sexual maturity at an early age are at increased risk of adopting disor-

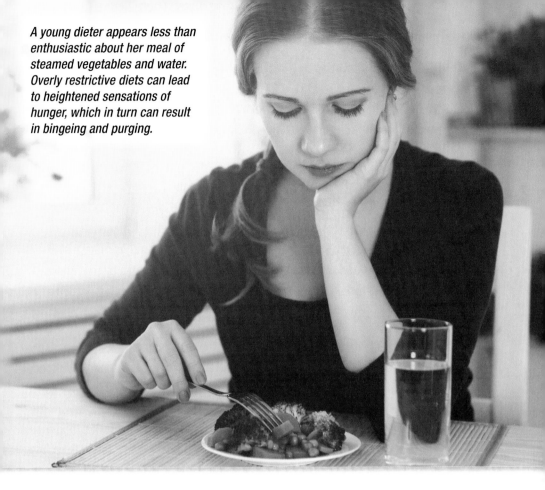

dered eating patterns. These young women fairly suddenly find themselves developing breasts, wider hips, and other physical signs of female adulthood. "They may wrongly interpret their new curves as 'being fat,'" ANRED states. As a result, they may

> feel uncomfortable because they no longer look like peers who still have childish bodies. Wanting to take control and fix things, but not really knowing how, and under the influence of a culture that equates success and happiness with thinness, the person tackles her/his body instead of the problem at hand. Dieting, bingeing, purging, exercising, and other strange behaviors are not random craziness. They are heroic, but misguided and ineffective, attempts to take charge in a world that seems overwhelming.[39]

33

Taught to Hate Their Own Bodies

In a moving narrative subtitled "My Battle and Recovery from Binge Eating Disorder," a young woman named Chevese tells how both she and her mother became prey to social pressures that contributed to their eating disorders. Chevese says, in part,

> I believe that my mother and I were predisposed to our journeys [to unhealthy eating habits]. Societal conventions taught us that the size of our bodies was not socially acceptable, though we were physically healthy. The message society sent us was that we must diet and diet often. My mother and I both struggled as children with weight issues and the stigma of bias by the media and society as a whole. We were taught early to hate our bodies and ourselves. Our self-esteem plummeted, and family strife soon entered our lives.

This series of events became the perfect recipe for developing an eating disorder, Chevese explains. As her weight continued to increase during her childhood, she steadily withdrew from friends and activities and came to rely on food for comfort. Her mother's alcoholism and her parents' divorce also took a toll, as did the alcohol and illegal drugs that Chevese herself started consuming. "But food was always the preferred substance," she continues. "I did my best to escape from [my troubles] through food. It was the only thing I could consistently rely on."

Quoted in Alliance for Eating Disorders Awareness, "Chevese's Story: My Battle and Recovery from Binge Eating Disorder." www.allianceforeatingdisorders.com.

Other Common Triggers

Medical authorities say that another common trigger for disordered eating is dieting. When a person goes on a reducing diet, especially an overly restrictive one, her or his body typically goes into survival mode. The body cannot think for itself, of course. It can only react to the stimuli the person presents it with. It does not realize that the sudden lack of food and nutrients it experiences is the result of its owner's conscious choice. Reacting as if that person is actually starving and in danger of dying, the body instinctually tries to get its owner to eat more by sharply increasing feelings of hunger. In most cases, the dieter eventually gives in to the gnawing hunger pangs and begins eating again, sometimes in the form of a binge. From there, fear of weight gain can lead to purging and/or starvation, behaviors closely associated with bulimia and anorexia. Still another kind of trigger that frequently leads to eating disorders consists of a simple yet disturbing remark made by a relative, friend, or even a stranger. That seemingly minor comment may tap into existing insecurities or worries that have already been bothering the person for some time. As a sudden trigger, the remark forces those troubled feelings to the surface. The person must then find some way to deal with them, and one way may be to turn to abusing food, naturally not realizing at first that it is abuse.

> "I believed that if I lost weight, I would gain control. I put all of my time and energy into becoming thinner. Before I knew it, my behaviors had become an obsession."[40]
>
> —Eating disorder sufferer Christina Neville

One young woman, Christina Neville, learned the hard way how much damage a single remark could trigger, saying that "for five years anorexia ruled my life." She continues,

I would think to myself, "Why I am I never happy in my life?" "Is it because there is something wrong with me?" Then an incident that started my eating disorder occurred. I was in a school play with some of my friends. At the time these were my first real friends and I thought I had to do whatever it took to fit in with them. But when I heard one of my close girlfriends at the time, behind my back, say that she thought I looked fat in my dress, it crushed me. I had always been comfortable with my weight and for my tall figure. But in that moment I made a connection in my head that, "Maybe this is why I'm unhappy. If I'm fat and other people think and feel that way, maybe I should change it." That summer I made the decision that I was going to lose weight, no matter what it was going to take. I believed that if I lost weight, I would gain control. I put all of my time and energy into becoming thinner. Before I knew it, my behaviors had become an obsession.[40]

Teens Are Particularly at Risk

These cases show that anorexia and other eating disorders have complex physical, emotional, and social causes. Doctors and other health professionals hope to gain a better understanding of these causes, and that can happen, they say, only through continued study of eating problems. They know that the more they learn about the causes of binge eating, bulimia, and anorexia, the more effectively they can treat these disorders.

The evidence is overwhelming that the dangers of these illnesses are especially acute for teens and other young people. Whatever the causes might be, psychologist Russo says,

> children showing problems in their early childhood are at higher risk for eating disorders later in childhood or adolescence. It is imperative that we catch signs and symptoms as early as possible. The potential consequences of an eating disorder in childhood and adolescence are profound and potentially more life threatening then developing one in later years.[41]

CHAPTER THREE

What Is It Like to Live with an Eating Disorder?

The life experiences of the millions of people who have had eating disorders are quite naturally extremely varied. After all, each person's family and social life is unique, and different people react to the ordeal of disordered eating in different ways. However, certain aspects of daily life, including the ways one reacts to and tries to cope with one's illness, are similar for most eating disorder sufferers.

Among these similarities are a constant preoccupation with food and one's disordered eating habits. Also common are various forms and degrees of emotional distress, which the sufferer typically tries to hide. As a teenager living with anorexia, for example, Shanel experienced both of these reactions to her disorder. "I couldn't go through a meal without knowing how many calories I was consuming," she recalls. Meanwhile, she found it harder and harder to deal with and contain her ragged emotions. "I was constantly sad for no apparent reason and would get angry very quickly," she says. In addition, "I completely isolated myself from my friends and family. . . . I was always feeling depressed. I was truly miserable."[42]

> "I completely isolated myself from my friends and family. . . . I was always feeling depressed. I was truly miserable."[42]
>
> —Eating disorder sufferer Shanel

Another reaction that most eating disorder sufferers tend to have is some level of denial that they are seriously sick. Former bulimic Mary Rowen, for instance, was aware that her eating patterns were seriously skewed. Also, she had heard that an eating disorder is a kind of mental illness characterized by self-destructive behavior. Yet, "despite the fact that I'd heard and read statements to that effect," she says, "I adamantly denied that I had a disease. After all, I couldn't be mentally ill. I wasn't psychotic, or self-destructive. I was just going through a 'phase.'"[43]

> "Years of my life had been consumed with a daily torture that I kept from everyone, especially those closest to me."[45]
>
> —Eating disorder sufferer Justin Shamoun

A Double Life

Thus, although individual family, school, and social situations vary, a majority of those who develop binge eating, bulimia, and/or anorexia share certain key feelings, experiences, and behaviors. Shame is one of the most common feelings. Mortified by their disordered eating patterns, they seek to hide their problem and to appear as normal and well-adjusted as possible. Everyday life for many sufferers, therefore, almost inevitably becomes a virtual tissue of lies.

Justin Shamoun, who developed his eating disorder as a young teenager, knows firsthand about the double life those with these conditions often lead. Until he entered the sixth grade, he had loved gym class, especially when the students would dive into the school swimming pool. But after his disorder took hold of his life, he remembers, "I would make up excuses as to why I couldn't participate, create lies as to why I couldn't swim that day, pretend I showered but hide in the bathroom instead."[44]

Later, as his body became overly thin from self-starvation, Shamoun put off his two-semester gym requirement until his senior year. His hope was that "eventually I would be what I considered acceptable, to take my shirt off in the locker room without being embarrassed." He never did feel confident enough about his looks, however. So in his words, "I learned ways to hide my body. This included making up fabrications as to why I couldn't go to events on days I thought I didn't 'look good enough' to be in public." Finally, Shamoun says, he reached a point at which

years of my life had been consumed with a daily torture that I kept from everyone, especially those closest to me. On the outside I was an outgoing, funny, nice guy that loved being around people. But this facade was fading as quickly as my grades were. It became too exhausting to lead this double life, and I didn't know where to turn.[45]

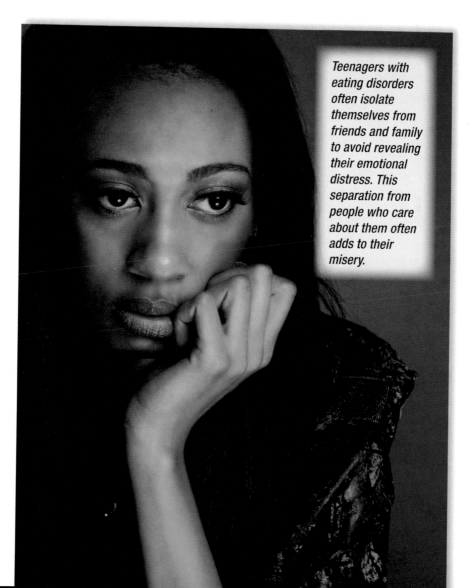

Teenagers with eating disorders often isolate themselves from friends and family to avoid revealing their emotional distress. This separation from people who care about them often adds to their misery.

Toward a New Personality

In some cases, the sufferer's constant lying can become so involved and complicated that she or he begins to take on a fake persona—in a very real sense an artificial personality. According to eating disorder specialist Dr. Judy Scheel, in creating the new persona, "some sufferers overcompensate." They may try to appear "overly self-confident and gregarious. They may act as if they have little or no concern for how others feel about them and appear to have very high self-esteem."[46]

Their real personality, however, harbors mainly the opposite feelings about their lack of control over their life. Beneath the phony façade they have created, Scheel explains, they are usually

> deeply worried about how others perceive them and acknowledge having very low self-esteem. They are painfully aware of the charade they play every day. Usually, the persona they have developed to conceal who they really are is not part of who they wish to be or how they wish to behave in life and relationships. Lies are used in order to protect themselves.[47]

Mental health experts recognize another kind of persona that some eating disorder sufferers use to deceive and manipulate those around them. These individuals are not haunted by and ashamed of lying to and misleading others. Rather, dishonesty has been a way of life for them "long before the eating disorder developed," Scheel points out. "As a result, the eating disorder is usually more difficult to treat. The persona they develop is unfortunately more ingrained and relied upon, often without conflict for them, i.e., they feel little guilt. They consciously do not believe they are compromising themselves or others."[48]

The Teeth and Stomach Are Under Attack

Beyond the lies they may tell others and/or themselves, most eating disorder sufferers inevitably wrestle with nagging, often painful physical problems as part of their daily routines. The many

A Male Bulimic's Story

Although eating disorders are more common among young women than young men, young men are not immune from developing these disorders. Estimates for the percentage of US males who suffer from eating disorders range between 2 and 5 percent. One study suggested that the proportion may be as high as 15 percent for gay men as opposed to 5 percent for straight men. One bulimia sufferer, Jack Harper, describes some of his personal experiences:

> For me, being a guy with an eating disorder was tough. I mean really tough. Sure, it's common for anyone with an eating disorder to feel ashamed or embarrassed. But, being a male with an eating disorder adds a whole extra layer of shame on top. If you were to look at the media, you probably wouldn't think that men got eating disorders. Even I thought it was just something that affected teenage girls (little did I know!). I felt a constant worry about anyone ever finding out that I was bulimic. . . . When I eventually did tell someone about my eating disorder my world didn't explode, I didn't suffer a heart attack, I didn't have a mental break down. . . . I felt relief, and that felt good. My eating disorder started when I was 23. I [soon found that] my will power was useless against the intense urges [I felt to binge and purge]. Eventually I would always give in. My life began to crumble. I transformed from an average, normal guy to an insecure, anxious, miserable mess.

Jack Harper, "How Being a Guy Stopped Me Getting the Support and Help I Needed to Recover from Bulimia." www.nationaleatingdisorders.org.

nasty and debilitating side effects of the repeated vomiting episodes undergone by bulimics are a clear example. First, when they regurgitate a recent meal, they bring up stomach acid along with the vomit. Over the course of weeks, months, and especially years, the acid damages the gums and teeth.

In particular, the acid tends to eat away the enamel that acts as a natural protection for the teeth. Unsightly discoloring and a steady rotting of the healthy dentin, the bony tooth tissue beneath the enamel, then ensues. "I won't even attempt to describe the damage I did to my teeth," Mary Rowen testified after bringing her rampant bulimia under control. "Instead, I'll tell you that over the past thirteen years, I've spent about seven hundred hours in the dental chair trying to repair that damage. (Yes, I've done the math.) Is this sounding glamorous yet?"[49]

The negative effects of the vomiting also frequently extend to the throat, esophagus, and stomach. Former bulimic Samantha Escobar recalls the pain and fear she felt after having binged and purged up to twice per day for many months. "I thought about it the same way some of my friends felt about yoga or meditation or face masks," she says. "It was just a part of my routine." In particular, she goes on, "there were these deep, intense stomach pains that felt like they were reverberating all over my stomach." Eventually, she says, "I started throwing up blood every few days. It wasn't just happening when I threw up on purpose. It would happen without any warning whatsoever after I ate any normal sized meal. My doctor said that my esophagus, having been weakened from years of wear and tear, was now more prone to ripping—thus the blood."[50]

> "I started throwing up blood every few days. It wasn't just happening when I threw up on purpose. It would happen without any warning whatsoever after I ate any normal sized meal."[50]
>
> —Former bulimic Samantha Escobar

Self-Induced Malnutrition

The adverse physical effects of anorexia can be even more severe than those for bulimia. First, people stricken with anorexia essentially starve themselves on a regular basis, which naturally causes their bodies to go into survival mode. As an anorexic consumes less and less food, she or he burns stored fatty tissues in an effort to make up for the lost calories. The result, of course, is that the sufferer gets increasingly thin.

If the anorexic behavior continues unchecked, eventually all fatty tissue will burn off and vanish. Nevertheless, the person's

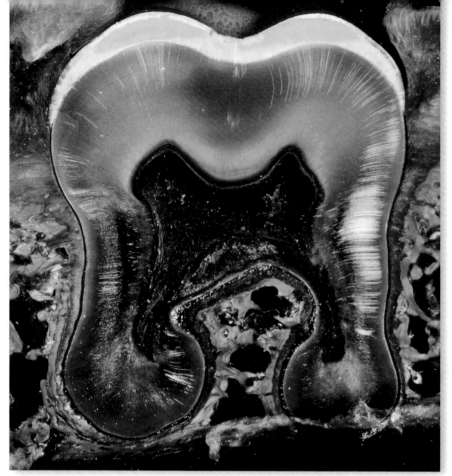

A light micrograph reveals enamel (bright gold) on a human molar. Stomach acid that reaches the mouth through repeated forced vomiting eventually eats away at tooth enamel.

body still needs various nutrients in order to continue functioning. To that end, it starts burning muscle tissue, and over time the muscles grow smaller, causing the anorexic to lose still more weight.

This process of starvation and loss of nutrients and body tissue is a form of malnutrition, a condition that normally occurs mostly in poor, undeveloped countries where there is not enough food for everyone. But whether it happens because of lack of available food or purposeful self-denial of food, the harmful physical effects on the body are the same and can make the everyday life of the sufferer extremely unpleasant.

Besides the steady loss of muscle tissue, a wide array of other detrimental symptoms of malnutrition can readily be found

From Tragedy to Hope

After Anna Westin died from anorexia in 2000 at age twenty-one, her family members decided to channel their grief into an effort to help other young people suffering from eating disorders. Led by Westin's mother, Kitty, they created the Anna Westin Foundation. In September 2002 the foundation opened the Anna Westin House in their hometown of Chaska, Minnesota. It was the focus of the first residential eating disorder program in Minnesota.

Anna's House, as most people called it, was a true community effort. Numerous people volunteered their time and talent or made regular donations, making the effort an overall success. In the following few years, hundreds of young women suffering from eating disorders received understanding and attention in Anna's House. Later, in the spring of 2008, the Westin family decided to make another major leap by merging the Anna Westin Foundation with a newer organization of the same type—the Emily Program Foundation. This move allowed the Westin family's existing outreach to expand and include many more young women in need. Today, Kitty Westin remains involved in these efforts by serving on the Emily Program's board of directors. The Emily Program Foundation comments that it "continues to work tirelessly to ensure that each individual and family impacted by eating disorders gets the support they deserve." In these ways, Anna Westin's tragic death was transformed into hope for thousands of fellow sufferers.

Emily Program Foundation, "History." http://emilyprogramfoundation.org.

among anorexics. They include low blood pressure, dry skin, thinning hair, low body temperature, delayed wound healing, and increased risk of infection (because of impairment of the immune system). Still other physical drawbacks of anorexic malnutrition are blindness, anemia (the loss of red blood cells, which makes it more difficult for the blood to carry oxygen to the body's tissues and organs), and heart problems.

Even when an anorexic experiences only some of these damaging physical effects of the illness, she or he becomes prone to fatigue and changes in mood and personality. According to Grainne Smith, an expert on eating disorders, for a person with severe anorexia "there is simply not enough energy available to keep up normal life as it was known before." Furthermore, an anorexic can find it harder and harder to hold on to friends and acquaintances. After all, Smith points out, "even talking takes energy." In addition, it is not unusual for an anorexic to find "it impossible to believe that anyone could love her or have an interest in her." Often she may begin "to sound irritable and bad-tempered over trivial things that never caused a problem before, and her perceptions of relationships and events change and distort as she loses the ability to think clearly and logically."[51]

Destroying Companionship

Evidence shows that this tendency to lose regular contact with longtime friends and acquaintances is actually one of the major lifestyle changes associated with eating disorders. As dietician and eating disorders authority Crystal Karges puts it, "While strong bonds may have once existed in a relationship, eating disorders encompass an overwhelming power to destroy companionship and fellowship."[52]

This parting of the ways can happen for a number of reasons. The most common reason is that people with eating disorders almost always retreat into their own separate, isolated sphere or living space. "Eating disorders are survival mechanisms, coping strategies for dealing with underlying issues that may be overwhelmingly difficult to face," Karges writes. Because of the difficulty in dealing with personal issues, sufferers often feel the effort will end in failure. To avoid embarrassment, they distance themselves from friends and even family members. Therefore, Karges explains,

> many eating disorder behaviors are done in secrecy, and the disease is perpetuated in isolation. It is not uncommon for eating disorder sufferers to begin avoiding social functions, and ultimately, relationships and loved ones, as they become more deeply embedded in the illness. Eating disorders become all-consuming, engulfing the individual struggling in negative thoughts and behaviors that harshly sever the most nourishing of relationships.[53]

> "Eating disorders become all-consuming, engulfing the individual struggling in negative thoughts and behaviors that harshly sever the most nourishing of relationships."[53]
>
> —Eating disorder authority Crystal Karges

As the person with the eating disorder retreats from once-normal activities and relationships, friends may react in different ways. Some may exhibit sympathy, understanding, and a willingness to do whatever is necessary to maintain the relationship. Others, however, may be unable or unwilling to expend the time and energy required to help their friend deal with the disorder. As a result, these friendships usually do not endure.

On the Outside Looking In

The amount of sympathy and understanding shown for someone with an eating disorder often depends on how close one is to the person in the first place. Family members and longtime friends are more likely to stick with the sufferer than are acquaintances. Typical is what happened to a young college student, who prefers to remain anonymous, after she developed bulimia and started purging and using laxatives almost every day. "My relationship with my roommates started to get really bad," she recalls.

> They told me at Thanksgiving that "we didn't click as roommates" and they didn't want to live with me next year. This really crushed me. I was blind to the tension I was causing in the apartment. [Still, I have come to believe] they are actually really not that nice and [that they] like to blame me for many things. [Eventually] they told me that my problem has made them develop their own body image problems, and that I am causing them.[54]

However, even friendship is not a guarantee of empathy and support. Another young woman who suffered from an eating disorder—Lindsey Avon—found herself abandoned by some close friends who, in her words, "were not supportive" of her predicament. "They didn't understand the disease or even try to educate themselves about it. Some people do not believe that an eating disorder is a disease. I have learned through years of therapy that I have to surround myself with good hearted, caring, positive people."[55]

These stories demonstrate that it is frequently hard to be on the outside looking in, and it can be equally difficult to know how to react. Karges, who counsels relatives of eating disorder sufferers along with the sufferers themselves, offers this advice to family and friends in such situations:

> On the outside, the vicious cycle of an eating disorder is frustrating and complex to understand. Watching someone you love slip into such dark shadows of despair is [painful], and it is even more difficult to feel as though you are unable to help. This can be true for friends as well as relatives. If your loved one is battling an eating disorder, you may feel as though your relationship has been replaced by this ferocious disease, or that the person you once loved is now unreachable. Know that there is always hope for recovery for the person in your life you care for, no matter how deep in their eating disorder they may be. Even though you may feel displaced in the relationship you once had, your continued presence in your loved one's life can make all the difference.[56]

Self-Inflicted Injuries

Karges and other experts say that, sadly, despite the ever-present existence of hope for recovery, some eating disorder sufferers reach a point where they give in to their despair. In that dark mental state, they may strike out at themselves in what the experts call an episode of self-injury. According to Eating Disorder Hope, such episodes consist of "a deliberate and direct injury or damage of body tissue, usually intended without suicidal ideation [thoughts]."[57]

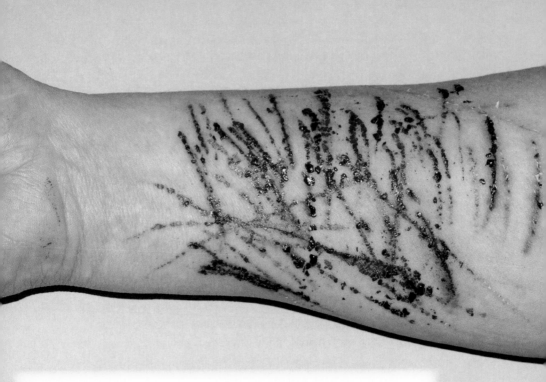

Cutting is a common type of self-injury seen in teens with eating disorders. Signs of cutting are usually most visible on the arms and legs.

The most common type of self-injury is cutting one's skin. It is most often done with a razor blade and concentrates on parts of the arms and legs. Other self-injury behaviors include scratching one's skin with fingernails, pulling out hair, burning oneself, ripping scabs from wounds, and eating or drinking toxic substances. Eating Disorder Hope states that sufferers most often employ these extreme measures in "an attempt to release anger, escape emotional pain, or in an effort to gain a sense of control."[58]

Family members and friends of those with eating disorders can look for the following familiar symptoms of self-injury: First, any fresh cuts, scratches, bruises, burns, or other wounds may be a sign. Moreover, if the person wears long sleeves or pants a lot, even in warm weather, she or he may be trying to cover up evidence of self-inflicted injuries. One or more broken bones can also indicate such behavior, along with the repeated excuse that the injuries were always the result of accidents.

A Fatal Step

Regrettably, some eating disorder sufferers end up taking a fatal step beyond self-injury. These individuals usually feel that their condition has totally ruined their life. Indeed, typically life seems miserable and hopeless to them and they feel that continuing to live with their illness is no longer realistic.

Experts on eating disorders are somewhat unsure about how many sufferers actually attempt suicide. A 2012 study by Florida State University researchers has been helpful in giving a rough idea. Of the college students with eating disorders who were interviewed for the study, an alarming proportion—more than a quarter—reported having a brush with suicide. More precisely, some 28 percent said that they had either experienced serious suicidal thoughts or had actually tried to take their own lives.

The study also ranked the three chief eating disorders as to how likely their sufferers were to have suicidal thoughts. Bulimia showed the highest rate of risk (45 percent), followed by anorexia (35 percent), and then binge eating (28 percent). These figures cannot predict exactly who among the sufferers of these conditions is going to consider suicide. Yet as Eating Disorder Hope points out, such studies are valuable in that they shine a light on the seriousness of the problem and serve as a reminder of how intertwined these disorders are with the dark thoughts that can lead to suicide. As the group notes, "Special attention is warranted for those struggling with eating disorders, as suicide ideations may be a daily part of their reality."[59]

Anna's Story

The story of one young anorexic—Anna Westin—illustrates how thoughts of suicide can become a regular part of a sufferer's daily life. A native of Chaska, Minnesota, she was born in 1978 and developed her eating disorder in her mid-teens. The illness came to consume her, as revealed in entries in her diary. "I am scared to death about what's going on right now," she wrote one day. "I can't have any control over my own mind. As much as I know what I need to do it's so hard to. My moods are very extreme. One minute I'll be depressed, then another, something will make me happy again."[60]

By the time she was twenty, in 1999, Westin's anorexia had become so severe that she required hospitalization. "What do I want?" she then wrote in her diary. "That is the most difficult question, when really I have two very conflicting answers. One [will] kill me, and at times this seems to be the most desirable." Westin lost her battle with anorexia when she took her own life the following year. The inscription on her grave marker reads, "In my end is my beginning."[61]

Westin's epitaph has proved prophetic. Her struggle and death inspired her family to create a foundation dedicated to helping other eating disorder sufferers to avoid her fate and achieve their own new beginnings. "I'm motivated by the loss of Anna and not wanting anyone to experience what she did, what we did," Westin's mother, Kitty, stated years later in 2015. There had been a lot of progress in battling eating disorders since her daughter's passing, she said. "There is a lot more awareness now and wonderful resources for people/families who are struggling. But we still need to do more."[62]

CHAPTER FOUR

Can Eating Disorders Be Treated or Cured?

Eating disorders can be treated using a wide range of techniques. However, experts on these conditions point out that even the most successful treatment cannot ensure a cure. This is because at present no known cure exists for eating disorders. Rather, the best that can be expected is that a sufferer will learn to manage the condition so that it no longer rules or disrupts daily life.

One reason that a complete cure is extremely difficult to find is that people with eating disorders are in a very real sense addicted to food—or more accurately, to abusing food. But unlike alcoholics and drug addicts, who do not need alcohol or drugs to live, people with eating disorders cannot escape from or give up the source of their addiction. Binge eaters, anorexics, and bulimics cannot simply give up eating since that would lead to starvation and death. Therefore, their only realistic choice is to learn to deal with food in ways that are as safe and healthy as possible. The fact that the sufferer must continue to consume the substance she or he has long been abusing makes both recovery and safely managing the disorder an extremely challenging goal. Nevertheless, recovery *is* possible as long as the person fighting the disorder is determined, courageous, and persistent. Former anorexic Kelly Joyce aptly sums up the most effective approach to recovery:

> I have learned that recovery is a process. It is more about balance than it is abstinence. Yes, abstinence from behaviors is a key component to recovery. But unlike drug or alcohol addiction, one cannot abstain from the very substance

that fuels our bodies, food. Recovery is about discovering a balance with food and a balance with life. It's progress, not perfection. Recovering is about learning to accept good enough NOW, not "if" or "when." When we start to accept ourselves for who we are and our bodies for what they are, we become free from the chains of our illness. Recovery is about courage. It is about the courage to take small steps, trusting that they will lead to great accomplishments. Recovery is about patience, compassion, and persistence.[63]

Inpatient and Outpatient Care

The several existing approaches to treating eating disorders fall into two general groups or types (which are used for both adult and teenage sufferers). One consists of attempting to physically repair and heal a body that has been ravaged by months or years of yo-yo dieting, bingeing and purging, and/or starvation. The other broad-based approach involves trying to heal the mental and emotional scars the patient has acquired during the fight with an eating disorder. This option is often called psychological treatment. The two general approaches are by no means mutually exclusive; often those who are helping the patient get better employ forms of both.

Of the various physical avenues to treatment and recovery, the one taken by those with the most serious and life-threatening cases of disordered eating is hospitalization. This approach has two principal forms—inpatient care and outpatient care. In inpatient care, the person remains in the hospital until the doctors and other health care providers feel it is all right for the patient to go home. In outpatient care, the patient lives at home but visits the hospital daily or even twice daily for a given length of time.

> "Unlike drug or alcohol addiction, one cannot abstain from the very substance that fuels our bodies, food."[63]
>
> —Former anorexic Kelly Joyce

The most severe eating disorder cases often require inpatient care. As a spokesperson for the Mayo Clinic explains, inpatient care is frequently necessary for people with anorexia who "are

Eating Disorders Research Is Poorly Funded

Although eating disorders affect an estimated 30 million US residents, or about 10 percent of the population, research into these disorders receives much less funding than other illnesses and conditions. According to the Academy for Eating Disorders, annual federal research funding for conditions such as alcoholism, schizophrenia, and ADHD (among others) is significantly higher than for eating disorders.

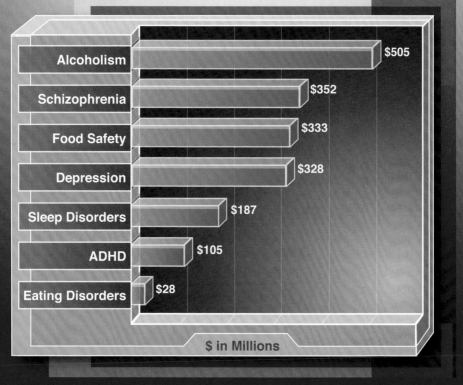

Category	$ in Millions
Alcoholism	$505
Schizophrenia	$352
Food Safety	$333
Depression	$328
Sleep Disorders	$187
ADHD	$105
Eating Disorders	$28

$ in Millions

Source: Academy for Eating Disorders, "Fast Facts on Eating Disorders," March 21, 2014. www.aedweb.org.

unable to eat or gain weight. Severe or life-threatening physical health problems that occur with anorexia can be a medical emergency."[64] Typical inpatient care includes force-feeding a person if need be, constant surveillance to be sure he or she does not binge or purge, and getting the patient back to a healthy weight. Once the individual's condition has improved enough and she or he is back to a healthy weight, the patient can usually switch over to outpatient treatment.

"Recovery Starts Within"

Eating disorder sufferers who have managed to recover are unanimous in saying that overcoming these illnesses is no easy thing. Former anorexic Odetta Kasa points out that much of what must change to spur recovery lies on the inside, in the mind and heart. Once she was able to turn her back on the emotions and fears that fed her disorder, she was on the road to success. "Recovery starts within," she begins.

> I realized that no one could help me better than I could help myself. I am still fighting. An eating disorder doesn't develop overnight, and it doesn't go away overnight. The feelings and emotions still linger, holding on for dear life, trailing along behind. But they will let go. They will let go when they realize that you're not paying attention to them anymore. They will let go when they realize that you're better off without them. They will let go when you do not give them a second thought, let alone a first. And finally, they will let go when you do not face them anymore. But the only way to not face them is to turn around, and at this point, the only way to move is forward. It's been a long journey, and a lot has changed over the years. I have faced my deepest fears and have discovered more about myself than I could have possibly imagined.

Odetta Kasa, "Nothing Happens Overnight," National Eating Disorders Association. www.nationaleatingdisorders.org.

Outpatient care is considerably more flexible than inpatient care for eating disorder sufferers, including teens. This is because outpatient care allows the patient to continue with the normal business of his or her life, including making a living and/or going to school. According to Eating Disorder Hope, young people, as well as adults, enrolled in outpatient programs typically meet with various types of heath care professionals "approximately 2–3 times per week. This level of care can be helpful to those who need to continue to work or attend school."[65]

Some eating disorder patients in outpatient recovery feel the need to visit the hospital every day, at least at first, and spend several hours in various forms of therapy. Those who put in this kind of major effort most often find that it pays off over time. A good example is the outpatient experience of a former teenage anorexic who identifies herself as Natalie C. "I was at appointments every day," she writes,

> and gradually lifted the veil that had been hiding life from me. It took me about a year to reach a healthy weight, and a healthy mindset. I worked on self-confidence and understanding that perfection is not possible. I learned to speak up and assert myself, and also how to listen. I learned a new form of control—how to understand my mind and body, and maintain the control I needed to keep both healthy.[66]

Another young woman who developed anorexia in her teens, Emma Demar, underwent both inpatient and outpatient treatment and says that she found them difficult but "tremendously rewarding." She reports learning "a great deal about myself that I will carry with me for the rest of my life. The strength and perseverance that enabled me to recover has made me even more confident in my ability to overcome any and all obstacles."[67]

> "I learned a new form of control—how to understand my mind and body, and maintain the control I needed to keep both healthy."[66]
>
> —Natalie C., a former teenage anorexic

Residential Care and Medication

Another overall physical approach to treating eating disorders is for the patient to attend a residential facility. Typically it is a house-like structure (or group of buildings) where a number of sufferers live together for a few weeks or months and receive twenty-four-hour care. Life in such a facility is most often fairly structured and scheduled. But one important goal is to provide the patients with the feeling of being in a comfortable home setting rather than a clinical hospital setting.

In a residential facility, a teenager or adult can focus on getting better while socializing with other people who are dealing with the same physical and emotional distress. The patients usually eat together and have ample opportunities to share their personal stories. Frequently this social interplay is helpful because long-time sufferers take heart in seeing that they are far from alone in their abuse of food. Patients follow specialized food plans, are regularly weighed, and undergo both personal and group therapy several hours a day.

The patients who attend residential facilities may also be involved with one of the chief physical approaches to treating eating disorders—selected medications prescribed by a doctor. Not everyone who suffers from these conditions needs to or should take these medications. They are administered by trained professionals on a case-by-case basis, and the individuals whose disorders are the most severe are the most likely to require them.

> "Antidepressants are the most common medications used to treat eating disorders that involve binge-eating or purging behaviors."[68]
>
> —The Mayo Clinic

Regarding this sort of drug therapy, the Mayo Clinic points out that "antidepressants are the most common medications used to treat eating disorders that involve binge-eating or purging behaviors." According to the clinic, an antidepressant may be especially helpful if you have bulimia or binge-eating disorder. Antidepressants can also help reduce symptoms of depression, anxiety or obsessive-compulsive disorder, which frequently occur along with eating disorders. You may also need to take medications for physical health problems caused by your eating disorder.[68]

Psychological Counseling

Whether treatment involves a hospital, a residential facility, or recovery at home, it also usually includes counseling of some kind.

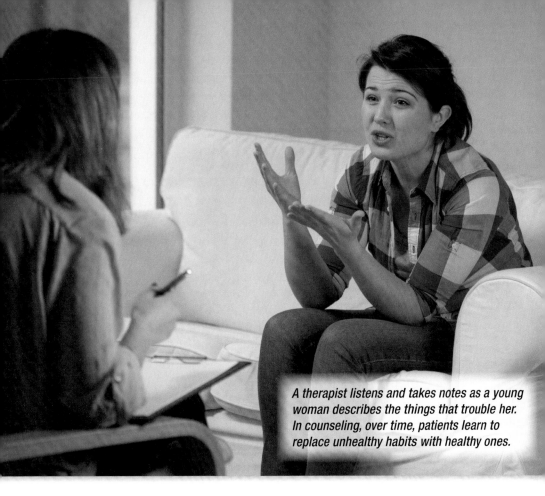

A therapist listens and takes notes as a young woman describes the things that trouble her. In counseling, over time, patients learn to replace unhealthy habits with healthy ones.

In fact, the Mayo Clinic makes clear, "psychological counseling is generally the most *important* eating disorder treatment. It involves seeing a psychologist, a psychiatrist who specializes in psycho-therapy, or another mental health counselor on a regular basis."[69]

In such counseling, the patient talks with the doctor or thera-pist about any and all issues of concern. Sessions can take place daily in hospital or residential settings or a few times a week in a doctor's or therapist's office. The purpose of the counseling is to teach the patient how to achieve both normal eating patterns and a healthy weight that can be maintained long-term. If the counsel-ing works, the Mayo Clinic states, the patient learns to "exchange unhealthy habits for healthy ones." Patients also learn to monitor their eating and moods and develop problem-solving skills. Addi-tionally, they learn to "explore healthy ways to cope with stressful situations."[70]

To achieve these goals, psychological counseling can take a number of different paths, and the doctor or therapist involved will choose the best one for each specific case. One of the most popular and useful treatments is cognitive behavioral therapy (CBT). Usually a fairly short-term treatment, it directly addresses specific behaviors, thoughts, or feelings connected to the eating disorder being treated. The goal is to help the patient to recognize the most potentially harmful thoughts and ideas that tend to trigger disordered eating behaviors.

CBT accomplishes that goal by breaking down the overall subject of the patient's disorder into smaller, more manageable issues. These may include various recurring emotions, feelings, or thoughts or typical physical sensations or actions associated with the food abuse. The counselor and patient talk about each issue separately, which helps the patient understand how it fits into the larger scheme of the eating disorder.

Another type of psychological therapy often used to treat eating disorders is dialectical behavioral therapy (DBT). The goal of DBT is to teach the patient to replace harmful coping methods with healthy ones. For example, the binge eater, bulimic, or anorexic may learn a more effective way of asking family and friends for help. Other coping strategies may include dealing with conflicts with relatives, finding better methods of resisting the temptation to abuse food, choosing between safe and unsafe behaviors, making oneself feel better about life without resorting to food abuse, and dealing with changing emotions.

Group Therapy

Such meetings between counselor and patient are often referred to as one-on-one sessions. This reflects the fact that the therapy almost always starts out in private and involves just those two principals. It is not unusual for patients who make significant progress in this sort of venue to emotionally connect with and come to rely on and even feel friendly toward their therapists. "My therapist Jane is one of the best people I've ever met," states former eating disorder sufferer Kat Watson.

The Healing Power of Poetry and Music

Art therapy, dance therapy, and equine therapy are not the only modern creativity-based treatments for eating disorders. Many teens, and some adult sufferers as well, have turned to writing, especially poetry (including song lyrics), to express themselves during the recovery process. During her long months of treatment, Emily Zahn, whose anorexia began when she was in her teens, used the exercise of writing poetry and song lyrics to help her purge what she saw as dark feelings haunting her soul. "I write poetry and music to help cope as I journey through recovery," she explains. "I think it is important for people struggling to find a passion or healthy outlet to share their stories and that is what I have done through my writing and music. I hope this inspires others to keep up the fight because health is beautiful and worth it."

Zahn adds that writing poetry and lyrics helps her express the strong humorous and playful side of her personality. "I am known for my humorous, sarcastic outlook on life," she says, "and I think that has proven as the strongest medicine for me. I do not look at my past experiences as sad or limiting, in fact I am quite proud of my ability to laugh at the endeavors that I have been through and make light of something that is so devastating for so many people."

Emily Zahn, "Regaining My Voice," National Eating Disorders Association. www.nationaleatingdisorders.org.

"When I visit her every month, we usually talk much longer than the allotted hour."[71]

However rewarding a person's one-on-one sessions may be, a majority of doctors recommend that sooner or later their patients move on to group therapy. This involves meetings in which a counselor moderates a discussion among four, five, or more individuals who have all suffered from the same eating disorder. Usually they get together one to three times a week and share their personal experiences and concerns while the counselor provides a larger context and offers helpful comments.

A number of different kinds of group therapy are at present employed to help eating disorder patients. One is family-based therapy, in which the patient's closest relatives sit and chat with him or her and the therapist. Family therapy is useful for all involved. It aids not only the patient but also the family members, who frequently gain new insights into their loved one's troubled thoughts and behaviors.

Still another type of group counseling consists of meetings of local support groups (also called peer support groups, fellowships, or mutual help groups). Existing in most American cities and towns, these are gatherings in which the members assemble periodically and share personal stories and information. Such meetings are quite often moderated by former eating disorder patients. But it is not unusual for a doctor or other health care professional familiar with disordered eating problems to sit in.

Other Kinds of Therapy

Several other types of treatment for eating disorders have developed over the years. One is nutritional therapy, which many doctors recommend as a supplement to one-on-one and group behavioral therapy. "Working with a registered dietitian should be incorporated in your treatment plan," says Crystal Karges in an article for Eating Disorder Hope. Karges points out that

> depending on the severity of your eating disorder behaviors and symptoms, you may meet with your dietitian in different settings, ranging from inpatient to outpatient. Your dietitian will work with you and your [treatment] team to address immediate concerns. Many dietitians will collaborate with your physician to determine any medical conditions that can be approached with nutrition therapy. This may involve reviewing current lab work or metabolic tests that may reveal nutritional deficiencies or problems.[72]

In addition to lab work, a dietitian will typically look at the person's complete medical history, any past tendency to go on reducing diets, any patterns of weight gain and loss, favorite foods used for comfort in the past, and relevant family history. In this specialized capacity, Karges explains, the dietician will

> guide you towards making peace with food and your body by making recommendations that can help you overcome challenges with food as well as normalize eating habits and behaviors. For example, if there are certain foods that you feel trigger you to binge, a dietitian can help you begin to [include] these foods by gradually incorporating them into your diet. A dietitian will also help you regulate your intake by recommending a meal plan that is tailored to your individual needs. This usually involves 3 meals per day and some snacks as appropriate with foods incorporated from all food groups to promote optimal nutrition.[73]

From Paints to Horses

Another approach to treating eating disorders—art therapy—originated as a tool for dealing with various mental disorders during the mid-twentieth century. But it was not seriously applied to eating disorder treatments until that century's last two decades. In an average art therapy session, patients may employ drawing, painting, sculpting, paper cutting, or other popular artistic media. Most often the counselor asks them to create an image or images that capture their inner feelings or thoughts. Then both counselor and patient discuss what the artwork means to the patient.

Another creative approach to treatment is dance or movement therapy. In this case, instead of expressing one's inner feelings and emotions through manual artistic media, one expresses them through body movements. The idea is for the patient to be able to use nonverbal means of conveying feelings. The counselor is trained to interpret certain movements in specific ways and

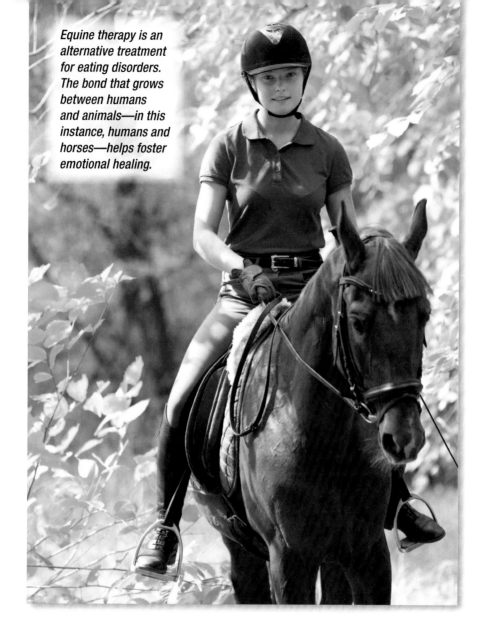

Equine therapy is an alternative treatment for eating disorders. The bond that grows between humans and animals—in this instance, humans and horses—helps foster emotional healing.

uses what he or she learns from the session to supplement data gained from the patient during other forms of therapy.

One of the newest forms of alternative treatment is equine therapy. As the term *equine* suggests, it employs horses. According to Eating Disorder Hope, it

is based on the premise that the bond that can grow between humans and animals will allow for emotional healing to occur. Activities that might be involved are care for and grooming of the animal and basic exercises guided by a horse specialist. Men or women who use equine therapy during treatment might have increased self-esteem and body image, particularly as the care for an animal has been shown to be an empowering experience.[74]

A Million Times Better

Whatever treatments eating disorder patients may undergo, most agree that they are ultimately helpful to one degree or another. Yet virtually all of those who have suffered from these destructive conditions concur that no matter how successful the therapy might be, recovery is still an extremely arduous process. "I won't sugar-coat it," Kat Watson says. "Recovering from the life I was living was even harder than living it in the first place. There were days I refused to get up, fun events I repeatedly skipped, and nights where crying myself to sleep seemed like the only option. But slowly, I got better."[75]

Another former eating disorder sufferer, Juliet Golden, agrees. As a teen she had a severe case of anorexia but was able to regain control of her life through hospitalization, followed by multiple forms of psychological therapy. "My eating disorder almost killed me," she says. "But it didn't." The reason she survived, she adds, was part-

> "There were days I refused to get up, fun events I repeatedly skipped, and nights where crying myself to sleep seemed like the only option. But slowly, I got better."[75]
>
> —Recovered anorexic Kat Watson

ly because of the excellent treatment she received at the hands of caring medical professionals. Also, she states, she reached deep inside herself to cooperate in the treatment, even when she felt she might not have the strength and energy to do so. In her words,

> After months in hospital, months of recovering at home, months in a Day Program which changed my life and years of therapy, I am alive. This is my greatest achievement,

because so many times, I could have given up, or my body could have given up for me. . . . My recovery is still a work in progress but I have solid foundations and am building up the walls, and with regular, adequate eating, skills, communication and love, one day I will be placing a roof over my head and locking the door so my Eating Disorder can never step foot near me again.[76]

Golden also emphasizes the need to be both brave and determined in order to get better: "I'm glad that all the times I just wanted to leave [the treatment program], I hung on. Because the life that you earn through recovery is a million times better than anything you could have expected, or dreamt of, or imagined for yourself."[77]

SOURCE NOTES

Introduction: "The Monster Inside Me"

1. Julie Saunders, "Road to Recovery," National Eating Disorders Association. www.nationaleatingdisorders.org.
2. Saunders, "Road to Recovery."
3. Saunders, "Road to Recovery."
4. Saunders, "Road to Recovery."
5. Saunders, "Road to Recovery."
6. Saunders, "Road to Recovery."
7. Saunders, "Road to Recovery."
8. Saunders, "Road to Recovery."
9. Saunders, "Road to Recovery."
10. Saunders, "Road to Recovery."

Chapter One: What Are Eating Disorders?

11. National Eating Disorders Association, "Get the Facts on Eating Disorders." www.nationaleatingdisorders.org.
12. John M. Grohol, "Symptoms of Binge Eating Disorder," Psych Central. http://psychcentral.com.
13. Grohol, "Symptoms of Binge Eating Disorder."
14. Quoted in Alliance for Eating Disorders Awareness, "Chevese's Story: My Battle and Recovery from Binge Eating Disorder." www.allianceforeatingdisorders.com.
15. Quoted in Alliance for Eating Disorders Awareness, "Chevese's Story."
16. Quoted in Alliance for Eating Disorders Awareness, "Chevese's Story."
17. Quoted in National Eating Disorders Information Center, "Battling Bulimia." http://nedic.ca.
18. Eating Disorder Hope, "Bulimia Nervosa: Causes, Symptoms, Signs & Treatment Help." www.eatingdisorderhope.com.
19. National Eating Disorders Information Center, "Clinical Definitions." http://nedic.ca.
20. National Association of Anorexia Nervosa and Associated Disorders, "Anorexia Nervosa." www.anad.org.

21. Quoted in National Association of Anorexia Nervosa and Associated Disorders, "Recovery: True Inspirational Stories." www.anad.org.
22. Quoted in National Eating Disorders Association, "Stories of Hope." www.nationaleatingdisorders.org.
23. Quoted in Alliance for Eating Disorders Awareness, "Jasmine's Story: My Battle and Recovery from Anorexia." www.allianceforeatingdisorders.com.
24. Quoted in Alliance for Eating Disorders Awareness, "Jasmine's Story."

Chapter Two: What Causes Eating Disorders?

25. Deborah A. Russo, "Toddlers and Tiaras: The Makings of Eating Disorders in Children," Eating Disorder Hope. www.eatingdisorderhope.com.
26. Russo, "Toddlers and Tiaras."
27. Palo Alto Medical Foundation, "Eating Disorders." www.pamf.org.
28. Quoted in National Eating Disorders Information Center, "Battling Bulimia."
29. Quoted in National Eating Disorders Information Center, "Battling Bulimia."
30. Eating Disorders Victoria, "Self Esteem." www.eatingdisorders.org.au.
31. Eating Disorders Victoria, "Self Esteem."
32. Samantha Goldberg, "Picture Perfect Memories," National Eating Disorders Association. www.nationaleatingdisorders.org.
33. Jackie DiVito, "Freedom and Strength," National Eating Disorders Association. www.nationaleatingdisorders.org.
34. Quoted in Marceia Rojas, "Social Media Helps Fuel Some Eating Disorders," USA Today. www.usatoday.com.
35. Anorexia Nervosa and Related Eating Disorders, "What Causes Eating Disorders?" www.anred.com.
36. Quoted in National Association of Anorexia Nervosa and Associated Disorders, "Recovery."
37. Arden Whitehurst, "Alive by Grace Alone," National Eating Disorders Association. www.nationaleatingdisorders.org.
38. Anorexia Nervosa and Related Eating Disorders, "What Causes Eating Disorders?"

39. Anorexia Nervosa and Related Eating Disorders, "What Causes Eating Disorders?"
40. Christina Neville, "Christina's Recovery Story: Embracing Perfection," National Eating Disorders Association. www.nation aleatingdisorders.org.
41. Russo, "Toddlers & Tiaras."

Chapter Three: What Is It Like to Live with an Eating Disorder?

42. Shanel Daudy, "Without Hope There Is No Progress," National Eating Disorders Association. www.nationaleatingdisorders .org.
43. Mary Rowen, "Talking Changed Everything," National Eating Disorders Association. www.nationaleatingdisorders.org.
44. Justin Shamoun, "Who Says You Have to Be Defined by Your Eating Disorder?," National Eating Disorders Association. www.nationaleatingdisorders.org.
45. Shamoun, "Who Says You Have to Be Defined by Your Eating Disorder?"
46. Judy Scheel, "Duplicity, Lies, Manipulation, and Eating Disorders," When Food Is Family (blog), Psychology Today. www .psychologytoday.com.
47. Scheel, "Duplicity, Lies, Manipulation, and Eating Disorders."
48. Scheel, "Duplicity, Lies, Manipulation, and Eating Disorders."
49. Rowen, "Talking Changed Everything."
50. Samantha Escobar, "Take It from Me: Don't Become Bulimic," TheGloss. www.thegloss.com.
51. Grainne Smith, Anorexia and Bulimia in the Family: One Parent's Practical Guide to Recovery. West Sussex, UK: John Wiley and Sons, 2004, p. 34.
52. Crystal Karges, "How Eating Disorders Can Affect Relationships," Eating Disorder Hope. www.eatingdisorderhope.com.
53. Karges, "How Eating Disorders Can Affect Relationships."
54. Roses1, "I Have an Eating Disorder," Experience Project. www.experienceproject.com.
55. Lindsey Avon, "There Is Always Hope: From a Wife's Perspective," National Eating Disorders Association. www.national eatingdisorders.org.
56. Karges, "How Eating Disorders Can Affect Relationships."

57. Eating Disorder Hope, "Self-Injury and Eating Disorders." www.eatingdisorderhope.com.
58. Eating Disorder Hope, "Self-Injury and Eating Disorders."
59. Eating Disorder Hope, "Suicide Risk Increased with Eating Disorders." www.eatingdisorderhope.com.
60. Quoted in PBS, "Perfect Illusions: Eating Disorders and the Family: Anna." www.pbs.org.
61. Quoted in PBS, "Perfect Illusions."
62. Quoted in Mollee Francisco, "Remembering Anna," *Chaska Herald,* August 6, 2015. www.swnewsmedia.com.

Chapter Four: Can Eating Disorders Be Treated or Cured?

63. Kelly Joyce, "The Courage to Heal," National Eating Disorders Association. www.nationaleatingdisorders.org.
64. Mayo Clinic, "Eating Disorder Treatment: Know Your Options, Part 2." www.mayoclinic.org.
65. Eating Disorder Hope, "Types of Treatment and Therapy." www.eatingdisorderhope.com.
66. Natalie C., "An Imperfect, Healthier, and Happier Adventure," National Eating Disorders Association. www.nationaleating disorders.org.
67. Emma Demar, "What I Learned in Recovery," National Eating Disorders Association. www.nationaleatingdisorders.org.
68. Mayo Clinic, "Eating Disorder Treatment: Know Your Options, Part 1." www.mayoclinic.org.
69. Mayo Clinic, "Eating Disorder Treatment: Know Your Options, Part 1."
70. Mayo Clinic, "Eating Disorder Treatment: Know Your Options, Part 1."
71. Kat Watson, "Inspirational Story," Eating Disorder Hope. www .eatingdisorderhope.com.
72. Crystal Karges, "Medical Nutrition Therapy for Binge Eating Disorder," Eating Disorder Hope. www.eatingdisorderhope.com.
73. Karges, "Medical Nutrition Therapy for Binge Eating Disorder."
74. Eating Disorder Hope, "Types of Treatment and Therapy."
75. Watson, "Inspirational Story."
76. Juliet Golden, "My Recovery: Rebuilding," Eating Disorder Hope. www.eatingdisorderhope.com.
77. Golden, "My Recovery."

RECOGNIZING SIGNS OF TROUBLE

Common Symptoms of Binge Eating
- Continuing to eat, even when full
- Hoarding food in order to eat it later in secret
- Eating normally in front of other people but overeating when alone
- Having feelings of stress or anxiety that can be eliminated only by eating a lot of food
- Experiencing emotional numbness or lack of sensation while overeating
- Never feeling satisfied one has eating enough, no matter the amount of food consumed

Common Symptoms of Bulimia
- Constant changes in weight
- Enlarging of the glands in the neck
- Suffering from an inflamed esophagus
- Often experiencing gastric reflux after eating
- Being suspected of using up large amounts of food from the refrigerator and cupboards
- Regularly eating in secret
- Experiencing a lack of control when eating
- Going back and forth between periods of overeating and fasting
- Frequently having to use the bathroom after meals

Common Symptoms of Anorexia
- Constant dieting even though one is extremely underweight
- Having an obsession with the calories and fat in one's food
- Eating by oneself and/or hiding one's food
- For women, experiencing the absence of three menstrual cycles in a row without being pregnant
- Suffering from depression or lethargy
- Feeling cold, especially in the arms and legs
- Hair thinning or loss
- Staying away from social functions, friends and family, and/or choosing to be by oneself a lot

The following organizations offer help for teens and others suffering from eating disorders, as well as detailed information about those disorders.

Binge Eating Disorder Association (BEDA)

637 Emerson Pl.
Severna Park, MD 21146
website: http://bedaonline.com

BEDA focuses on providing information about the prevention and treatment of binge eating disorder (BED) and the associated stigma of being overweight. The organization offers education, outreach, counseling, and helps those with eating disorders find proper diagnosis and treatment.

Emily Program Foundation

1295 Bandana Blvd. West, Suite 210
St. Paul, MN 55108
website: http://emilyprogramfoundation.org

The foundation provides support for people with eating disorders and expands community awareness of these conditions. Also, the group endeavors to make sure that eating disorder sufferers and their families receive proper support.

National Association of Anorexia Nervosa and Associated Disorders (ANAD)

PO Box 640
Naperville, IL 60566
website: www.anad.org

ANAD focuses on prevention of eating disorders and educates and helps people who need to find treatment and support. ANAD has a helpline, school outreach programs for children and teens, prevention programs, and support groups across the nation.

National Eating Disorders Association (NEDA)
165 W. Forty-Sixth St., Suite 402
New York, NY 10036
website: www.nationaleatingdisorders.org

NEDA offers programs and services that provide support for people with eating disorders and their family members.

National Eating Disorders Information Centre (NEDIC)
200 Elizabeth St.
Toronto, ON M5G 2C4
website: http://nedic.ca

NEDIC focuses on fostering awareness of what eating disorders are, preventing them, directing sufferers to proper treatment, and offering the public extensive information about these disorders.

National Institute of Mental Health (NIMH)
6001 Executive Blvd., Room 8184
Bethesda, MD 20892-9663
website: www.nimh.nih.gov

The agency's mission is to expand people's understanding of mental illnesses, including eating disorders, by performing medical research that might lead to prevention or even a cure.

Renfrew Center Foundation
475 Spring Ln.
Philadelphia, PA 19128
website: http://renfrewcenter.com

With seventeen locations nationwide, the Renfrew Center helps both adolescent girls and women who suffer from eating disorders to reorder their lives in positive ways, all in hopes of eventual recovery.

UCLA Eating Disorders Program

150 UCLA Medical Plaza
Los Angeles, CA 90095
website: http://eatingdisorders.ucla.edu

The UCLA Eating Disorders Program at Resnick Neuropsychiatric Hospital for more than thirty years has offered treatment services that are gauged to the individual needs of children, adolescents, and adults who suffer from eating disorders.

Books

Elizabeth Bellenir, ed., *Eating Disorders Information for Teens.* Detroit: Omnigraphics, 2013.

Lee W. Blum, *Table in the Darkness: A Healing Journey Through an Eating Disorder.* Downer's Grove, IL: IVP, 2013.

Brittany Burgander, *Safety in Numbers: From 56 to 221 Pounds, My Battle with Eating Disorders.* Tucson AZ: Wheatmark, 2016.

Carolyn Costin, *8 Keys to Recovery from an Eating Disorder.* New York: Norton, 2011.

James Lock, *Help Your Teenager Beat an Eating Disorder.* New York: Guilford, 2015.

Christine Wilcox, *Teens and Body Image*. San Diego: ReferencePoint, 2016.

Christine Wilcox, *Teens, Nutrition, and Dieting*. San Diego: ReferencePoint, 2016.

Internet Sources

Alliance for Eating Disorders Awareness, "Brenda's Story: My Battle and Recovery from Anorexia." www.allianceforeatingdisorders.com/portal/brendas-story.

Eating Disorder Hope, "Binge Eating Disorder: Causes, Symptoms, Signs, and Treatment Help." www.eatingdisorderhope.com/information/binge-eating-disorder.

Eating Disorders Foundation, "Prevention of Eating Disorders." http://eatingdisorderfoundation.org/learn-more/about-eating-disorders/prevention.

FamilyDoctor.org, "For Parents: Eating Disorders in Teens." http://familydoctor.org/familydoctor/en/teens/food-fitness/tips-for-parents-weight-and-eating-behavior-problems-in-teens.html.

Angela E. Gambrel, "Determined to Die? Suicide and Anorexia Nervosa," *Surviving ED* (blog), HealthyPlace, September 15, 2012. www.healthyplace.com/blogs/survivinged/2012/09/determined-to-die-suicide-and-anorexia-nervosa.

Crystal Karges, "How Eating Disorders Can Affect Relationships," Eating Disorder Hope. www.eatingdisorderhope.com/treatment-for-eating-disorders/family-role/how-eating-disorders-can-affect-relationships.

National Eating Disorders Association, "Binge Eating Disorder." www.nationaleatingdisorders.org/binge-eating-disorder.

National Institute of Mental Health, "Eating Disorders Among Children." www.nimh.nih.gov/health/statistics/prevalence/eating-disorders-among-children.shtml.

Palo Alto Medical Foundation, "How the Media Affects Teens & Young Adults." www.pamf.org/teen/life/bodyimage/media.html.

Deborah A. Russo, "Toddlers & Tiaras: The Makings of Eating Disorders in Children," Eating Disorder Hope. www.eatingdisorderhope.com/treatment-for-eating-disorders/special-issues/toddlers-tiaras-the-makings-of-eating-disorders-in-children.

INDEX

Note: Boldface page numbers indicate illustrations.

Academy for Eating Disorders, 53
American Academy of Child and Adolescent Psychiatry, 23
Anna Westin Foundation, 44
anorexia
  association with suicide, 49
  distortion of body image and, 17–19
  health risks of, 20–21
  mortality rate for, 10
  progression of bulimia to, 16–17
  risk of suicide among sufferers of, 49
  symptoms of, **11,** 69
Anorexia Nervosa and Related Eating Disorders (ANRED), 32, 33
antidepressants, 56
art therapy, 61
athletes, as vulnerable to eating disorders, 26–27
Avon, Lindsey, 46–47

binge eating/binge eating disorder
  association with suicide, 49
  bulimia *vs.*, 15
  as gateway to more serious eating disorders, 10, 15
  risk of suicide among sufferers of, 49
  symptoms of, 10, **11,** 12,69
Binge Eating Disorder Association (BEDA), 70
body image
  distortion of, 16–19
  low self-esteem and, 24, 26
  social trends/media and, 29, 34
body mass index, 13–14
Boone, Pat, 13
boys/men
  binge eating among, 10
  eating disorders among, 9, 18, 27
  suffering from eating disorders, personal experiences of, 38–39, 41
bulimia, 10
  association with suicide, 49
  health risks of, 40–42
  personal account of sufferers of, 15, 41
  on impacts on personal relationships, 46
  risk of suicide among sufferers of, 49
  shame associated with, 15–16
  symptoms of, **11,** 16, 69
bullying, 28

calories
  amount consumed by binge eaters, 12

obsession with, 26, 69
Canadian National Eating
Disorders Information Centre
(NEDIC), 15, 71
cognitive-behavioral therapy
(CBT), 58
coping mechanisms
eating disorders as, 24, 28
replacing harmful methods
with healthy, 58
withdrawal from social
relationships, 45–46
cutting (self-injury), 48, **48**

dance therapy, 61–62
dehydration, 16
Demar, Emma, 55
depression, 9, 23
dialectical behavioral therapy
(DBT), 58
diet industry, 29
dieting, 13
as trigger for eating disorders,
34–35
DiVito, Jackie, 28

Eating Disorder Hope, 16, 28,
47, 48, 49, 54
on equine therapy, 62–63
eating disorders
age and risk for, 9
among young men, 10, 18,
27
causes/risk factors for
perfectionistic attitudes,
30–32
school-related pressures,
26–28, 30–32
social trends/media, 29–30
deaths from, 9–10

emotional distress associated
with, 37
false personas assumed by
sufferers of, 40
health risks of, 9, **11**
anorexia, 20–21, **21,** 42–45
bulimia, 16, 40–42
information sources on,
70–72
personal accounts of
sufferers of, 4–7, 15, 38–39,
41
personal relationships
impacted by, 45–46
prevalence of, 8
public awareness of, 13
recovery from, 51–52
personal accounts on, 7,
51–52, 54, 55
research funding for, *vs.* other
conditions, **53**
treatments for
art therapy, 61
dance/movement therapy,
61–62
equine therapy, **62,** 62–63
goals of, 51
group therapy, 58–60
inpatient, 52–53
medication, 56
nutritional therapy, 60–61
outpatient, 54–55
prevalence of people with
eating disorders receiving,
9
psychological counseling,
56–58, **57**
triggers for
bullying, 28
dieting, 29, 34–35

negative remarks, 4
  puberty, 32–33
  See also specific disorders
Eating Disorders Victoria, 24, 26
Emily Program Foundation, 44, 70
equine therapy, **62,** 62–63
Escobar, Samantha, 42
esophagus, effects of vomiting on, 42

fashion models, 29
Florida State University, 49

gender
  prevalence of eating disorders by, 8
  as risk factor for eating disorders, **25**
  use of unhealthy weight-control behaviors and, 9
Golden, Juliet, 63–64
Grohol, John M., 12
group therapy, 58–60

Harper, Jack, 41
health risks, 9, **11**
  of anorexia, 20–21, **21,** 42–45
    as life-threatening, 52–53
  of bulimia, 16, 40–42

inpatient care, 52–53

Joyce, Kelly, 51–52

Karges, Crystal, 45, 47, 60, 61
Kasa, Odetta, 54

laxatives, 20, 27
  health risks from, 16

malnutrition, 42–45
Mayo Clinic, 56, 57
  on causes/risk factors for eating disorders, **25**
men. *See* boys/men
mortality rate, for anorexia, 10
movement therapy, 61–62
music, as creativity-based treatment, 59
Mysko, Claire, 30

National Association of Anorexia Nervosa and Associated Disorders (ANAD), 9–10, 18, 70–71
National Eating Disorders Association (NEDA), 8, 10, 18, 27, 71
National Institute of Mental Health (NIMH), 9, 71
Neville, Christina, 35
nutritional therapy, 60–61

O'Neill, Cherry Boone, 13
osteoporosis, 20, **21**
outpatient care, 54–55
overweight/obesity
  body mass index and, 13
  as result of binge eating, 12

Palo Alto Medical Foundation, 23
poetry, as creativity-based treatment, 59
psychological counseling, 56–58, **57**

puberty, as trigger for eating disorders, 32–33
purging/vomiting, 16
health risks of, 40–42

recovery
   from eating disorders, *vs.* cure for, 51–52
   personal accounts on, 7, 51–52, 54, 55
Renfrew Center Foundation, 71
research funding, for eating disorders *vs.* other conditions, **53**
Rowen, Mary, 38, 42
Russo, Deborah A., 22–23, 36

Saunders, Julie, 4–7
Scheel, Judy, 40
self-esteem, 19, 23, 34, 40
   equine therapy and, 63
   negative body image and, 24, 26
self-injury, 47–48, **48**
Shamoun, Justin, 38–39
Smith, Grainne, 44–45
social media, 30
Starving for Attention (O'Neill), 13
stomach, effects of vomiting on, 42
suicide, 49–50

teeth, **43**
   effects of vomiting on, 41–42
treatment(s)
   art therapy, 61

dance/movement therapy, 61–62
equine therapy, **62,** 62–63
goals of, 51
group therapy, 58–60
inpatient, 52–53
medication, 56
nutritional therapy, 60–61
outpatient, 54–55
prevalence of people with eating disorders receiving, 9
psychological counseling, 56–58, **57**
triggers, of eating disorders, 32
   bullying, 28
   dieting, 29, 34–35
   negative remarks, 4
   puberty, 32–33

UCLA Eating Disorders Program, 72

vomiting/purging, 16
   health risks of, 40–42

Watson, Kat, 58–59, 63
websites, promoting eating disorders, 29–30
weight
   obsession with, 18
      among student athletes, 26–27
   use of unhealthy behaviors to control, 9
Westin, Anna, 44, 49–50

Zahn, Emily, 59

PICTURE CREDITS

ABOUT THE AUTHOR

In addition to his numerous acclaimed volumes on ancient civilizations, historian Don Nardo has published several studies of modern scientific and medical discoveries and phenomena. They include *Vaccines*, *Teens and Birth Control*, *Breast Cancer*, *The Deadliest Dinosaurs*, *The Scientific Revolution*, and *Gender Identity Disorder*. Nardo, who also composes and arranges orchestral music, lives with his wife, Christine, in Massachusetts.